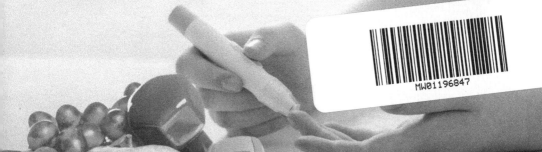

A Diabetic's JOURNEY

A Memoir

LUCY ANA KRASNO

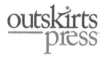

This book is dedicated to my mother Grace as well as my grandmother Anastasia both of who suffered from diabetes, and to all of those who struggle each day to battle this unforgiving disease. I hope each reader will better appreciate the importance of support from family and friends and the critical role parents and caregivers play in helping diabetics manage their disease and not allow it to define them. My journey with diabetes is shared with millions of others; together we are stronger by sharing our experiences and supporting efforts for continued research for a cure.

TABLE OF CONTENTS

PREFACE

In 1921, Canadian physician Frederick Banting discovered insulin. It was a breakthrough at the time for those who were diagnosed with diabetes.

In 2019, nearly 100 years later, there are over 400 million people with diabetes worldwide, many of whom are undiagnosed. Millions more are pre-diabetic, have insulin resistance or metabolic syndrome which can lead to chronic diabetes. Diabetes has become an epidemic and can lead to serious disability and several related health problems. In many cases it has led to heart disease, blindness, amputations, kidney failure, and neuropathy.

Globally, diabetes treatment costs are approaching two trillion dollars each year. Today, due to medical advances and specialized care, diabetics have more choices for managing their condition effectively and with good self-care, are able to live long productive lives.

My story is just one of millions who are suffering on a daily basis battling diabetes. I am a survivor.

Chapter One

An Early Diagnosis

My name is Lucy and I have an autoimmune condition called Diabetes Mellitus Type 1. As I write this story, I consider myself fortunate to be alive and thriving. Like many others, my diagnosis at the age of three changed the course of my life's journey and yet, I have managed to create a good quality of life and learned to accept what my condition requires.

I was born in Trenton, New Jersey and I was the first member of my extended family to be born in the United States. My mother was born in The Ukraine and did not come to this country until 1958. Her family left Eastern Ukraine in 1943 during World War II and traveled throughout Europe as refugees until they settled in a refugee camp in Austria. When World War II ended in 1945, my maternal grandfather applied to come to the United States, however, at that time the country was not accepting immigrants. My grandfather then applied to Brazil; his family of seven was accepted and they settled on a farmstead and went to work. After three years, they moved to Sao Paulo, Brazil for better job opportunities. Sadly, in 1954 my grandfather passed away in a tragic accident where he was hit by a truck while riding his bicycle to work. At this time his five eldest children (one being my mother) went to work full-time to support the family. My mother was only 14 when she got a job in a factory and went to night school with her older brother, Jaroslav. In 1958, her brother Alex applied to come to the United States. My grandmother Anastasia corresponded by mail with her family in The Ukraine and found out that her nephew Misha had come to the United States from Germany. Misha sent my mother's family a visa to enter the country. On arrival to the United States, my mom met a man who was a friend of Misha that would ultimately become my father. He had arrived in the country a few years earlier and was also Ukrainian. In 1959 they were married.

In 1961, my mother was excited to welcome me into the world as a healthy baby girl. She checked me thoroughly – I had all five fingers and all five toes. My mom's family came to visit me in the hospital, and all were overjoyed. Sadly, my uncle Jaroslav found my father in the hospital parking lot in his car with his door ajar and his arm hanging out of the door, nearly falling out of the car. He was passed out drunk. My father's whereabouts were unknown when my mother went into labor. Who knew at that time how this would impact me throughout my life.

The three of us lived in a one-bedroom apartment on the first floor of a building that had previously been a bar. There was no phone or washer and dryer, and any phone calls were made with a payphone down the street. My mother said I was a good baby, never cried much and was always smiling. My father was a full-blown alcoholic. He got up in the morning, went to work, went to a bar after work, and drank. He often left my mother and I alone, would come home drunk every night, then continue drinking and frequently start an argument. My mother left her job as a timekeeper to take care of me and my father was angry that that she stopped working. Many times, he would threaten my mom and throw things. When I was six months old, the situation between them was worsening. One night he came home and smashed the TV. Another time, he broke the fish tank creating an enormous mess. My mother told him many times that if he ever got physically abusive, she would leave him. One night he came home very late and my mother was beside herself. She was home alone with me and I was asleep. An argument erupted over his drunken state and my father punched her in the stomach very hard. She immediately took me, left everything behind, and walked to my grandmother's house. My grandmother was terrified for us and said we could stay as long as we needed to. The next day she returned to our apartment with a police officer to pick up our things as she was terrified what he might do next. When they came to the apartment, he had changed the locks. The policeman broke in and my mom packed what she needed for me and a few things for herself. My mother had made up her mind to leave my father for good, but money was going to be tight. She contacted a lawyer, but he wanted way too much money to file for divorce. The lawyer had suggested $25.00 per month for child support, but my father refused to pay, and told her he would never give her a divorce. She did not pursue the payment because she could not afford the lawyer.

My father visited me a few times at my grandmother's house, and she was in fear for her life. We were still living in New Jersey, and that was the only time he came to see me. He never paid any support and was not able to show it if he had a heart for me.

After two years, the extended family decided to move to the Midwest and my mother determined that we would move also. We arrived in a new apartment flat in Chicago in 1963, and my mom decided to work any minimum wage job to support me. She knew how to sew – a wonderful skill she learned when she was a teenager growing up in Brazil. She got a job sewing at a factory making pockets on men's suits and overcoats. The job was piecework, the faster you made the pockets, the more you got paid. The job was steady, and she worked there for 7 years taking the bus every day. Her employer offered health insurance for she and I, but only for hospitalization.

As a toddler my life was normal – playing outside with neighborhood kids, drawing in coloring books, playing with toys. I got a hold of some chocolates one time and my uncle Jaroslav, who was also my Godfather, took a picture of me after they smeared chocolate on my face to capture a great photo. Little did I know what my future held for me and chocolate. My mom did not have a driver's license and depended on my uncle to drive us where we couldn't take the bus. We got to know new people through our church, and we were lucky to have my grandmother and my uncles for support. My mother's side of the family had close friends that were a large part of our lives as I was growing up.

Because my mom was working all the time, she decided to take me on a fun outing to an amusement park called Riverview in Chicago. I was still young, but we saw lots of interesting things and despite my mom's hesitancy, we rode the roller coaster. It turned out to be a bit more than we bargained for and my mom held me incredibly tight and was extremely scared. We got off the ride and my mom was shaking. Later, when I was older she told me she wished she had never taken me on that ride and I often wondered if that event may have had something to do with my developing diabetes.

Around my third birthday in 1964, I started developing some strange symptoms. As a matter of fact, I can still remember my mother's concern after noticing I was losing weight, had no appetite and started to wet the bed at night. I had become lethargic and clearly lacked the energy of a normal toddler. My mother quickly suspected something was very wrong when one day after work my grandmother told her I was urinating very frequently and had an unquenchable thirst – wanting to drink water constantly. We made an appointment with a doctor my uncle recommended who was an older man in his late 50's and we were instructed to bring in a urine sample. The doctor examined me, gave me an injection (of what, we do not know) and told my mother I would be okay and that I did not need to come back for a follow up. He made no mention of the urine test, so we don't know if it was even checked. That evening I wet the bed again which had become an almost daily occurrence. Instead of getting better, I was getting worse.

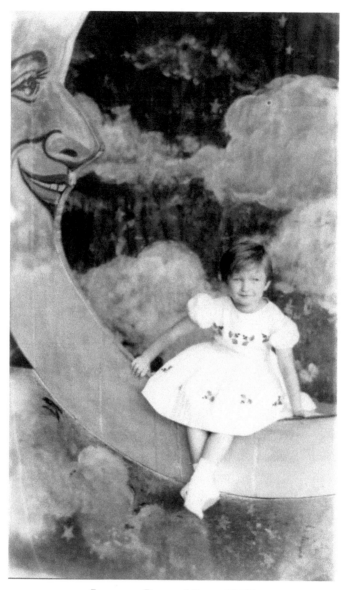

Lucy on Paper Moon 1964
Before Diabetes Diagnosis

Two weeks later, my mom was getting ready to go to work, and had to catch the bus. She did not want to disturb me as I slept and simply kissed me on the cheek and left. During her break, my mom called my grandmother, Anastasia to check on me. My grandmother told her that I still hadn't awakened, and that I was breathing heavily. My mother rushed home immediately, taking two buses to get there. She called my uncle Alex (who lived upstairs) to drive us to the hospital. My mom hurriedly carried my limp, unconscious body to the emergency room. The emergency room staff took me right away and started asking about the symptoms I had and whether anyone in my family had diabetes. My mom had never even heard of diabetes or what it even meant. They then asked my mom to sign a medical consent form so they could perform a spinal tap. Frightened, my mom gave her consent— all she wanted was for me to wake up.

Although my family did not understand this, I was in a diabetic coma. I had all the classic symptoms – frequent urination, unquenchable thirst, weight loss, no appetite and lethargy. In about an hour the results came back from the spinal tap and the young intern told my mother I had Diabetes Mellitus Type 1. This diagnosis was going create a profound change in our lives. My mom asked the doctor if I was going to live. I was running a very high temperature of 105 degrees and was lying on a bed of ice in my diaper. He answered that he did not know. My mom cried and started to pray. She was in shock and disbelief. I was only three years old, a baby, and she was terrified. My mom stayed with me at the hospital day and night and did not sleep or care to eat. After the third day at the hospital, my grandmother came to give my mom some relief. My mom took the bus home, kneeled by the bed where I slept and prayed to an icon of the Virgin Mary. She prayed for the Virgin Mary to please heal her daughter knowing that the Virgin Mary had lost her son. Later that day, my mom took two buses back to the hospital. She came into my hospital room and within the hour I opened my eyes and said "I'm hungry and I want a scrambled egg". I still remember that moment and how happy my mom was. At that point I had no memory of where I had been or why I was in the hospital.

I stayed in the hospital for four more days for monitoring and lowering my blood sugar back to normal levels. I was on an IV insulin drip and after three days I finally ate a complete meal. My appetite was back. The nurses started to give me insulin injections daily and for a three-year-old this was scary and very difficult. I cried each day with every injection. I had to start on a diabetic diet to keep the blood sugar under control. Imagine a three-year-old child needing to be on a diet! I was placed on 1200 calories and every portion had to be weighed by grams on a scale. If I had too much food and too little insulin, my blood sugar would go up creating hyperglycemia. If I had too much insulin and not enough food, I could experience a dreaded insulin reaction creating hypoglycemia. Either situation could result in death.

Once I came home from the hospital, our new lifestyle had to begin. My mom had to learn how to give me injections every morning. I would scream at the top of my lungs. The injection would burn after going in and I would rub the spot to make it feel better. This was very hard and confusing for a three-year-old who was thinking, why is my mom hurting me? I thought she loved me. It took a long, long time for both of us to get used to this new routine. After my mom left for work, my grandma had to comfort me and calm me down until the pain went away so she could give me breakfast. A diabetic always needs to balance the insulin ratio with the amount of food given. A lot of the time I did not want to eat everything. My grandma struggled every day to get me to eat what I needed. Frequently, I would open the refrigerator door to see what I could grab. I remember this one time when my grandmother opened the freezer and I saw a box of chocolate chips. I asked if I could have some and she said "no honey, you can't right now." Sugar was not for me. Being the only diabetic in the house was very hard for me. I felt so cheated when I couldn't eat the delicious things they were eating. My uncles who were in high school at the time, always ate a lot when they came home. I saw popcorn, sandwiches, peanuts, RC Cola, and I couldn't have any of it. I didn't understand why I got yelled at when I tried to eat something that I wanted.

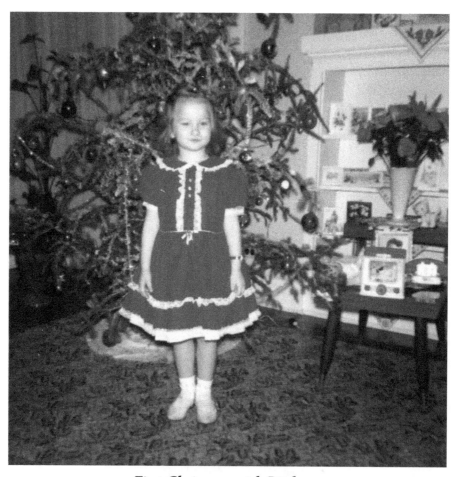

First Christmas with Diabetes

In order to maintain my blood sugar levels, my grandma needed to feed me at the same time every day. She used to cry because she knew if I didn't eat, I would end up in the hospital again. She used to pray to God in front of me so that the Lord would give me the strength to eat on time. I would eat eventually, but it was not easy for me. Afterwards, I would go on with the rest of the day playing with toys. Barbie dolls were my favorite and were the first friends I had. They kept me occupied so my grandma could do the cooking, laundry, cleaning, and keep an eye on me.

My mom was constantly worrying about me while she was at work. She would call my grandma during every break. I know my condition put a great deal of strain on the family, but looking back at family photographs I noticed I always had a smile on my face. I felt secure living in a home with several family members, even though they were not my siblings. After dinner everyone would relax in the living room and we would watch TV shows until it was time for bed. In the summertime we would spend time in the backyard after dinner.

After a while, I started to become more active. My insulin was working and I had a lot of energy. We lived in a two-flat, and my uncle Alex, his wife and baby lived upstairs. I used to run up and down the stairs full of curiosity. Eventually my activity was catching up with me. Along with not always eating a full breakfast, I started to have insulin reactions - low blood sugar. One morning after not eating enough, I had a very bad reaction. At the time I was just four years old. I recall my head felt strange and my vision started going black. It was fading and I could barely see anything. I screamed to my grandma, "I see monsters, I see monsters!". My grandma knew to give me ginger ale or sugar cubes. She held me in her arms and said "drink, and then chew." I followed instructions because I just did not feel well and would do anything to make it go away. Back then there was no way to predict glucose levels in the blood, but it was clearly too low.

During those years we used a testing kit that would show how much sugar was in the urine but even if it was negative, there was no way to establish a number. Eventually I started to come back to normal. My vision was coming back and I was feeling better. My grandmother held me and said, "no more monsters, no more monsters, shhh, it's alright. Baba is here, nothing will happen to you." Baba is Ukrainian for grandmother. She rocked with me until I could get up. This was my very first experience with extreme low blood sugar, and I still remember it over 50 years later.

I did have more insulin reactions, although they were not as severe since my grandma was vigilant about my eating. She used to say – "eat Lucy, chew Lucy." She would sit and watch me until I finished everything. Now that I was more active, if I wanted something to eat between meals, I could. On one particular occasion, I remember eating cottage cheese and applesauce. I could actually eat it instead of just looking at it. Eventually, my mom bought me some coloring books to keep me occupied, and I used to love to color in them. I would color in the living room while my grandma read the newspaper or cross-stitched in between doing housework. I was so fortunate to have such a loving grandmother who could care for me.

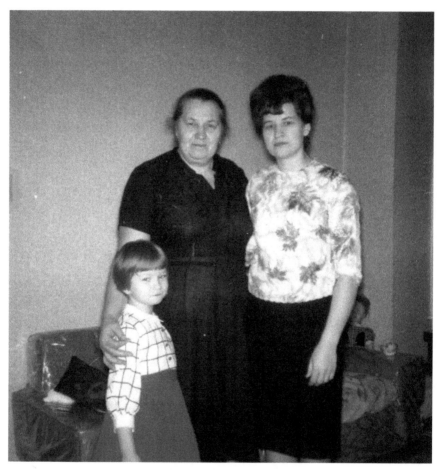

Lucy, Baba and Mama 1965

The day finally arrived when I could start school. Like many kids, my first day of kindergarten was traumatic for me. My mom took me to sign me up for the first day of school. I gripped her hand when I walked into the room. As I walked to the teacher, Mrs. Fox, I started to cry and whimper and hold on to my mom, because now I knew she was going to leave me with this strange new woman that I didn't know anything about. Mrs. Fox greeted me very nicely, took my hand, and told me that she was going to be my kindergarten teacher. I can still remember her blond beehive hairdo and light-colored glasses. My mom started to tell her that I was special because I had diabetes, and she brought a little pencil case filled with sugar cubes and some apple juice in case I needed it. My mom had to leave to go to work, and I started to cry a little bit, but then I settled in with Mrs. Fox and the rest of the class. Starting school, I did not speak any English because my grandma spoke to me only in her native Ukrainian. Mrs. Fox had called everyone to get their blankets to sit on the floor and she was going to read us a story. All the children sat down, and I followed. Mrs. Fox read several stories and then started showing us the alphabet on the board. Before I knew it, school was over and my grandma was waiting outside to pick me up. I was so happy to see her and hugged her with my little arms around her legs. We walked home hand-in-hand, and I started telling her about my exciting day at school.

I looked forward going to school the next day. Each day was a fun, new experience and I hardly ever thought about my diabetes, insulin injections, or eating. I started to learn the alphabet and made some new friends. By now the insulin injections were an everyday part of my life and although I didn't look forward to them, I knew they were a necessity. I must admit, my grandma still had to coax me to eat as breakfast was not my favorite meal.

The very next week Mrs. Fox started to offer new activities in class. Slides, jump rope and more – these were all fun and new to me. Baba came to pick me up after school and I was so excited to tell her about my experiences. Kindergarten went by quickly that year and I enjoyed making friends in the neighborhood and at school. I even remember I had a little boyfriend named Kevin that was in my class and lived nearby. We sometimes held hands as we walked home from school. He had a variety of pets that he would bring over including a duck, a rabbit, a hamster, a puppy, and a kitten. Kevin would come over with other kids and we would all do coloring books together in the living room. Baba had a Polish lady friend from the neighborhood with a daughter named Pasha that used to stop by and talk. I became friends with Pasha too, and I felt like I was starting to get popular! I didn't think about being a diabetic anymore. Although I always knew I had to take my medication and make sure I ate lunch on time, I enjoyed that I just got to be a kid and could focus on other things..

Chapter Two

—————

School Days With Diabetes

Autumn came and I started first grade. My new teacher, Mrs. Conlon, taught us how to read and write, and we also started learning to do simple arithmetic.

I used to carry a small purse to school to keep my sugar cubes with me. I remember being the only one in my class who had a purse. I would hang my purse on the metal fence in the schoolyard so I could play hopscotch, jump rope, run around or do other activities. One day, I saw another girl go into my purse to see what was in it but she didn't take anything. She asked me why I had sugar cubes in my purse, and I said they were for an emergency. She didn't pursue it any further. Since I couldn't have sugary things for breakfast like Frosted Flakes, I had to have a scrambled egg with toast or liverwurst spread on bread which I didn't like very much. I would pretend to eat it, but instead sneak it out of my mouth into a paper towel or napkin and throw it away when Baba wasn't looking. This wasn't a good idea for a child on insulin. One day right before recess, I started to feel funny. My insulin was kicking in hard from not eating all my breakfast. My body had too much insulin floating around and inadequate food to work on in my body. I needed some sugar, otherwise I would faint. I felt dizzy and when the recess bell rang, we had to walk down two flights of stairs to get to the playground. I remember walking along the wall of the stairs by the hand rail and hanging on to it. I had my purse with me on my shoulder. I had grown rather tired of always taking my purse with me and I often left it in the classroom, but that day I took it with me. As I walked down the stairs, my vision was fading and I was in the beginning stages of a severe insulin reaction. As we got outside to start recess, I hung my purse on the fence and got several sugar cubes from my purse and quickly started to eat them. After I finished eating, a girl came up to me and wanted to know what I was eating. My hands were shaking, I was sweating, and I felt faint. I could hardly stand up and I was in and out of dizziness. I ignored her as I continued to eat and swallow, but she was curious and did not go away. The girl kept asking me what I was eating, and I became angry and said in a loud voice "Nothing!!" I stood by the fence, mostly to hold myself up. My mom and Baba were not there to rescue me. I had to deal with this episode by myself, and I did. I soon started talking with my classmates, then the bell rang. Darn it! Diabetes got in the way! An hour later, I went home to eat lunch. Baba always had a nice wholesome meal for me. That day, I remember having minestrone soup and rice topped off with some fruit. I can't remember whether I'd told her about my hypoglycemic incident. I walked back to school for the rest of the afternoon. This was now a way of life for me. Up and down blood sugar. I was so active all the time. If I wasn't doing homework, then I was running around outside looking for the next activity. After school I would get together with some girls from the neighborhood and we would jump rope and then have contests to see who could jump for the longest time. I had to do the best, of course! So, I was using up my blood sugar constantly.

As the school year went on, I started getting a lot of infections in my throat. I was six and a half years old at this time. My mom was constantly spending money on me for doctor visits. I remember I had a very good pediatrician who was also very gentle. His attitude was always positive about my diabetes when speaking to my mom and encouraged her to let me be myself and that I could participate in any activity I wanted. In a year's time, I had over 20 throat infections. All the money my mom made working overtime in the factory went toward my medical costs and medication. I started to miss school quite often and was getting behind. The doctor told my mom my tonsils were getting very bad and they needed to come out. Being a diabetic, constant infections were hard on my body especially when combined with a high fever. It seemed like the right decision to have my tonsils removed.

It was wintertime when I was admitted for the surgery and had to stay overnight. The nurses hooked me up to an IV the night before and tried to explain to me that they had to stick a needle in my hand. I was scared, but I didn't show it. I just nodded my head and said ok. I felt the needle go in and it did indeed hurt. My mom and Baba were not there. Here I was alone to deal with another scary thing.

When I woke up from surgery, my mom was there along with my Godfather for support. Shortly thereafter they rolled in a cart with ice cream. It was such a treat to be able to eat something with sugar and cream without restrictions. Now I didn't feel so bad about the surgery! My throat was painful and it was hard for me to swallow for a long time. The diabetes made the healing process take much longer. It took about a year for that weird feeling in my throat to go away and it felt like I was missing something. My mom needed to closely monitor my diabetes during this time and adjust my insulin. Baba also checked my sugar levels in my urine by using the Clinitest kit with the activated tablets. My mom and grandmother were my personal home nurses, always following my diabetes and supporting me. They were my angels. I remember starting to feel better and not experiencing throat infections, so the surgery was definitely necessary.

Time passed and I started going to school again. I was now in second grade. I had a new teacher and new classmates. I made friends very quickly with a girl named Penny. We sat next to each other at the same desk and giggled, made notes and tried to pay attention to the teacher. We were always doing something that had nothing to do with schoolwork. Sometimes playing tic-tac-toe or some other game. One time the teacher asked the class who they thought were their best friends. Penny told everyone I was her best friend! After that I gave her a hug and I was so happy.

Penny was turning seven years old and her mom was throwing a birthday party for her. She gave me a handwritten invitation. I ran home from school and showed Baba, "look, look I was invited to a party!" telling her with glee. I was so excited, my first birthday party! I told my mom I needed to buy a present for Penny. Mom agreed and we bought her a game. My mom always worried about me, especially so with me going to a party, what I would eat and how I would feel. I told her I would be alright. I really wanted to go, but I didn't know what to expect. This was my first party and my mom drove me to Penny's house. I remember having so much fun – we played games, Penny opened presents, and everyone had cake. My mom had told me not to touch anything with sugar in it, but what did I know? Cake was cake. I'm sure I had some. We were so active running around, I'm sure it didn't affect me much. The party lasted a few hours and I remember talking about it for days.

I walked to school every day by myself unless the weather was bad, then I got a ride. About a block from my house the patrol boys were on duty protecting us while crossing the street. There was a small bush that grew by the corner and these boys used to drop things in that bush. When I walked by, I would find all sorts of things they carelessly dropped including pennies, small toys and even a quarter once. The kids at school told me about the corner pharmacy down the block that sold penny candy and gum. My friends and I walked there from school during recess. My favorite candies were Jolly Ranchers watermelon sticks and Lemonheads. This new endeavor felt sneaky, but I went along. My mom and Baba didn't know I went there. I also used to find loose coins that my uncles' left on a dresser. I would take them to go and buy bubble gum and candy. I would stash my candy in a certain dresser drawer for when I wanted something sweet. At one time I had accumulated so much candy that it almost took up half the drawer. One day, when my mom was in the bedroom looking for something, she opened the drawer and discovered all my candy. Her jaw dropped and she demanded to know where I got all of it. In a coy voice, I told her I was buying it at the pharmacy. I knew I was going to get scolded, and I did. She immediately took all the candy away from me. I cried but I knew sugar was forbidden for me. No longer were loose coins left lying around the house. Baba and mom used to send me to the local grocery store sometimes to pick up a gallon of milk or bread. It was a block away and I walked there alone frequently. They wanted me to be like the other kids that went for small errands. As you entered the store there were several bubblegum machines in the entrance of the store. If I was lucky to find a penny, I would buy a piece of gum when I went there. I didn't need to tell anyone and that little treat made me happy.

Occasionally Baba would buy me some barbeque potato chips and I would have those or a piece of cheese after school when I could run and play outside. Those snacks were a luxury. Other kids would have them and not think twice about balancing it out with insulin, but this was always on our minds.

One day I must not have eaten a lot for either breakfast or lunch. It was mid-afternoon, I came into the house and wasn't feeling well. I couldn't talk well. As suggested by the doctor, my mom gave me ginger-ale right away to treat my low blood sugar. That afternoon I felt worse than usual. I couldn't pronounce words and had a hard time speaking. My uncle Oleg gave me a child's book to read aloud. I had a hard time remembering how to pronounce anything and it took me several minutes to get the words out of my mouth. He told me to keep trying and I wanted to try but it was very difficult. The low blood sugar had severely affected my brain. Even though I was eight years old I was still horrified about what was happening to me. Why couldn't I remember how to read? There are many types of insulin reactions that present different symptoms, but this one was intense. After drinking a lot more ginger-ale, I finally regained some clarity and started to read normally. Uncle Oleg got me to laugh and smile and helped me to come back. My mom called the doctor and told him about the incident. He told her that she did the right thing and explained that this can happen with severe low blood sugar.

I always wore a pendant that identified that I was a diabetic. On the back it had my name and phone number. I used to hide it under my clothes when I was at school. I didn't want anyone to ask me about it because I didn't really know how to explain diabetes, or want to, I just wanted to fit in with the rest of the kids.

The summer passed and school was back in session. That September I went on my very first field trip to a museum in downtown Chicago. I was a bit scared but I knew I would be with my teacher and all my friends from school. That day I went to school with my purse and sugar cubes inside, my diabetic pendant and my lunch. Baba made sure I had a sandwich, some juice and a banana. I was ready for anything, all bases were covered. Baba warned me, "make sure you eat everything in your lunch bag during the lunch hour when you break!" Even at my age I had come to know that if I omitted eating something and we did a lot of activity I could have low blood sugar and my teacher would be stuck with the situation.

We arrived at the museum, a huge building that was so exciting for us. We walked through many interesting displays and before I knew it, we were taking a break and sat down to eat our lunches. I wasn't really hungry yet, but I opened my lunch bag and took out the sandwich and hardly had time to finish before the teacher asked us to finish up and get in line. Everyone rushed to throw away their lunch bags and move on. I did the same. I suddenly realized I had thrown away my banana, and that Baba had reminded me to finish everything! I ran to my teacher and said, "I didn't eat my banana" and started to cry. I wanted her to find it in the garbage. She tried, but there were so many bags in there that looked the same she was unable to find it. I panicked. What would happen to me since I didn't eat my banana? I tried to enjoy the rest of the day, but I was full of anxiety. Luckily, I didn't experience any low blood sugar symptoms at all. It was one o'clock, and time to head back onto the bus to go back to school. The teacher didn't seem too concerned that I had unintentionally thrown away my banana, my potential lifesaver. I reflected her attitude and I calmed down as well. This was a sign of the times – lack of awareness or understanding by teachers and the critical role of food in a diabetic situation. I was on my way back home, so all would be well. I came home and told Baba the story. She shook her head from side to side and was thankful that nothing happened to me. My mom heard about it later that night. That was probably my first frightful experience away from home, and I still remember it like it happened yesterday. It taught me an important lesson to follow directions for managing my diabetes no matter what.

My mom took me in for my usual doctor visit. In the room on the table was a copy of the Children's Bible. Since I frequented the office so much, I always liked to see that book and look at the pictures and then ask my mom about the stories. Mom saw that I really enjoyed the book and bought me my own copy. Baba always taught me prayers at home, even though I didn't really know much about what I was saying. I had my first communion, so I knew several prayers by heart, and I had to practice them. One afternoon I was sitting on the front porch and I was quietly going through the book and looking at the blue sky. My little cousin who lived upstairs was coming down the stairs, he was about three or four years old. As he came down the stairs he yelled in his little voice "Lucy is a diaper-betic, Lucy is a diaper-betic," over and over. I got up and ran into the house. I didn't want to be a diaper-betic!! Even at that age I felt so insulted. What did I do to deserve this? He was making fun of my diabetes. But the diabetes was not mine, I didn't want it, I was merely stuck with it. I told Baba what happened, and she assured me not to worry.

Like most moms, mine was always looking out for my welfare, and wanted to talk to the doctor about how to make my life easier. It was always very difficult for my mom to give me injections. She was weary of being the bad guy because she knew that it hurt. I remember having deep pits in my arms and legs from the needles because I didn't like to rotate my injection sites. I had learned early on that when an injection is given repeatedly in the same area the tissue becomes desensitized and the pain is less severe. My young arms and legs looked like pitted mounds on the moon. The doctor suggested that I could and should learn how to give myself injections and presented the idea of going to diabetes camp. The first suggestion was scary and the second was worse. We worked with a nurse at the hospital that showed me how to draw up a syringe the right way and then inject into the orange. Despite my fear, I went home and practiced on an orange a few times. I simply refused to be my own pin cushion. I told my mom I couldn't do it and I didn't want to. She tried pushing me a bit, but then backed down. Instead she said she would send me to the diabetes camp where I would be with a lot of other children and I could learn how to give injections there. She reassured me that there would be adult counselors there for any problems or emergencies. It would be for the summer, and since there would be other children, she somehow thought it would be fun. Fun? What could be fun about being with a bunch of strangers with diabetes? How could I be away from home, away from my mom and Baba and all my friends and relatives? This was not like I was going away to college, this was diabetes camp and there was nothing about it that was even remotely appealing to me. How would they know what I needed, and what kind of food I had to have? There was no use fighting it, my mom already made up her mind and I had to accept my fate.

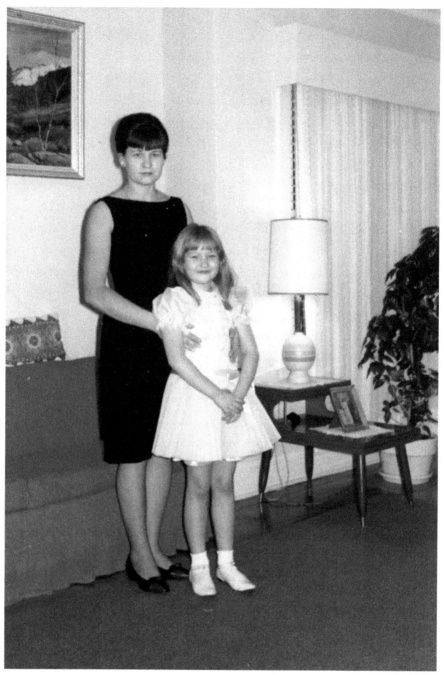

Lucy and Mama 1968

She was filling out the forms for "camp" and had them ready to mail with the payment. I was full of fear about being alone in a strange place. In a final attempt I said, "mom I don't want to go" and she said, "you are going." My pleas continued for the next 20 minutes. I got so red from crying and protesting the idea that she finally gave in to me. I lit up. "I don't have to go?", "No", she said, "you don't". Right or wrong, I had won. As you can imagine, I skipped out of the room and I didn't bother her for the rest of the day. I was ecstatic!

During this same year, I started to have pain in my lower calves. They felt very tight and I could not put my heels on the floor to walk. I tried very hard, but I had to walk on my tiptoes to move. I saw the doctor and he decided to put me in the hospital and run some tests. Shortly after I was admitted, the doctor brought in a specialist to see me. He did several tests including pricking my legs with a long thin needle to see if I had any sensations. He could not determine what was causing these symptoms, and he did not find any abnormality. I was also scheduled for an EEG to check my brain waves. The nurse put sticky tape ends on my head and connected some electrodes and then gave me a sedative so I would relax. I was very nervous, and I didn't want to sleep. I was fighting it, I didn't like what they were doing. It turned out that she could not finish the test because I could not relax. After a few days in the hospital, I was released and sent home. Since I had difficulty walking, Baba had to carry me on her back from one room to another, usually from the living room to the bathroom, if I needed it. It took a long time for the tightness to go away until I could put my heels on the floor and walk normally. One day the symptoms were gone and I was able to take a step again. The cause of this was never determined and I was just happy to be able to run around again.

At the next doctor visit we were introduced to a new magazine called, *Diabetes Forecast*, published by the American Diabetes Association. It focused on recent developments in diabetic care, stories about diabetics and a way to contact other people with diabetes by writing to them. A few weeks later the first issue came in the mail. Under the magazine title, I remember there was a picture of Mary Tyler Moore. I knew her! She was on the Dick Van Dyke Show. She had diabetes? And, she's a movie star. Wow, I didn't know there were diabetic movie stars! I was happy to see that she and I shared something so awful. Though it wasn't anything to *really* be happy about, it reminded me that I was not alone. Someone famous had this too! Mary Tyler Moore became the spokesperson for diabetes at that time and she became my inspiration. I would have been honored to meet her - it felt oddly comforting to know that someone famous was dealing with this disease just like I was.

I was encouraged to see her story and continued to read the issues that came in the mail. Reading new information about diabetes opened my eyes about the disease. As it turns out, diabetes was much more than just injections and not eating sugar. I learned about carbohydrates and how they were like sugar to the body, the food pyramid, and more about symptoms of high and low blood sugar levels. It was all coming together.

I was starting to understand diabetes from other sources other than my doctor and my mom.

One issue came with a red cover and on the front page it said in bold letters, *Diabetes; Leading cause of Blindness, Kidney Failure, Amputations*. I was shocked! I was only nine years old. I ran to my mom in panic and said, "look mom, look what this magazine says! Diabetes can cause all of this!" She had a look of horror on her face as well but in a reassuring voice said, "don't you worry about this." How could I not worry? I had diabetes. Would that headline be my future? I don't think she knew how to handle what the magazine cover said. Maybe she didn't want to believe it herself. Was I going to go blind? This was way too much for a nine-year old to face. How could this happen to me? I really began to hate having diabetes and it became a curse word. Oh, how I hated that word! It made me wonder if I was even going to live very long, my young mind was troubled.

At my next doctor visit, my mom questioned the cover of the magazine. The doctor just smiled and said, "don't read those things and don't worry about it." Eventually, I was able to see that the magazine was providing information to people to make sure they took care of themselves so these things didn't happen to them. After that, my mom made a point of hiding that magazine from me so I couldn't find it anywhere in the house. In time, I forgot about it and my childhood continued.

That winter, I was bored after school one day. I wanted something to read so I went through the local phone book as Baba was reading a newspaper about events in her homeland Ukraine. I was going through the pages and I stumbled on the "F" section where I saw funeral homes. Reflecting on all the scary things I'd read, I started to think about funeral homes and dying. I had already been to a funeral for a 13-year old girl a few years earlier who died of a heart problem. I remember her young face as she lay in the casket and thought about how she and her sister had come over to my house to play in my bedroom. Although her funeral didn't seem to bother me at the time, it did start me thinking about death. I also wondered what would happen if I lost a parent. When my mom came home from work, I asked my her, "What would happen if I lost a parent, would I be a half-orphan?" She just looked at me funny. "Why would you want to know that? I suppose you would be a half-orphan," she said. She then asked Baba why I was asking those questions. She didn't know, but it all tied back to what I found in the phone book.

A few days later, Baba got a long-distance call from my aunt on the East Coast. She had just heard the news from a friend at her church that my father had passed away. Baba gave the phone to my mom and she talked to her sister. Aunt Nadia said he was in the hospital several days prior and all she knew was that he had lost a lot of blood.

Mom decided we were going to the funeral and in just a few days we were on an airplane. My Godfather, Jaroslav had dropped us off at the United Airlines terminal which was going to be my first flight ever. I remember the stewardess had given me peanuts for a snack and I asked my mom if I could have the whole packet, and she said it was ok. We met my aunt and uncle at the airport and drove to their house where we stayed for a few days.

That first morning after arriving we started to unpack and get ready for the wake. Later that day we drove to the funeral home and I could see that my mom was a nervous wreck. Sensing that made me nervous, too. My uncle on my father's side met us by the door. My mom hadn't seen him in years and the next thing I knew my uncle asked to take some pictures of me. He kept taking one right after the other. My mom noticed that I had a fearful look on my face so she pulled me away.

As we walked into the next room, my hands were like ice. I was petrified and didn't know what to expect. I just remember seeing big beautiful flower arrangements and my grandmother, whom I didn't even know, sitting there waving a handkerchief on her face while sobbing. As I walked in, the funeral director told her I was her granddaughter. This was the first time she had seen me since I was an infant. She was very overweight and yelled in a loud voice, "Oh Lucy!" I was already a little scared and that scared me even more. Who was this woman I'd never met before? Why was she yelling those things? She came over and hugged me so hard it hurt and then started kissing my face. She wouldn't let go and I didn't like it. This was a stranger to me and I remember the funeral director actually had to tear her off of me. I was very startled and didn't know what to do. She yelled to me "I have so much to give you! I have so much for you!" I didn't care, I didn't know her, and it meant nothing to me. My mom grabbed my hand and walked over to the casket where I saw and essentially met my father for the first time. He was dead at 34 years old. Why was I meeting him for the first time like this? My mom put her hand on his cold hand and then said a prayer as we kneeled by the casket. I did the same following her lead. I understood he was my father, but I never knew him. He had never tried to contact me while he was alive. For some reason my mom thought it would be good for me to see him this way. I didn't agree. I had felt cold all over my body the entire time we sat near the casket. My mom didn't want to talk to my grandmother at all due to the way they had treated her when I was an infant.

Looking back, I don't think we were at the wake for more than an hour. My mom didn't show it at the wake, but she was deeply suffering emotionally. My mom made me hug my grandmother and tell her we were leaving. My grandmother kept yelling at me, "he loved you so much!" Her words meant nothing to me, and it just made my mom more upset. We left the building and got into my aunt and uncle's car and started driving away. My mom's hands were shaking and her heart was beating fast. I could feel her anxiety. She started to talk to my aunt angrily. "How could she tell my daughter that her father loved her so much! He never even tried to contact her at all during those nine years! No child support, no nothing! Not even a birthday present!" I heard all of the conversation, and as any child would do I concluded that my father didn't care about me. As a nine-year old, I didn't know how to process this, it all came about so fast. We arrived at my aunt's house and got ready for dinner. My aunt was a good cook and always made a generous meal. Soon it was bedtime and we slept in her guest room on twin beds. My mom kept sighing, she was reeling by the whole day and thinking about what was said at the wake. Each hour that night my aunt's coo-coo clock chimed and as the night progressed the clock sounded more macabre. I don't know how either of us slept after that chilling day. Somehow, I did get some sleep, and soon the sun came up and it was morning. Mom told me to get dressed because we had to be on time for the funeral. I know I must have had breakfast, but don't remember what I ate. Diabetes was still there, and I had to eat and take my insulin. It was a chilly day. We arrived and I saw my grandmother in the front pew along with her sons and their wives along with my cousins Kelly and Laura. Everyone was crying. They actually knew my father. I didn't. We sat in the row behind them. Shouldn't I have been in the front row? I was holding my mom's hand. This day was different. Everyone was paying attention to the church service and I was in back of them. When the church service ended, the family members paid their last respects to my father. The casket was open and I approached it with my mom. I felt numb and cold. I stared at him for the last time. In that moment I questioned, did I look like him? I couldn't decipher either way. I put my hand on his hand and, of course, my camera-happy uncle captured that moment. He probably felt this was the one and only time any of them would ever see me. And as it turned out, it was true. Others followed to pay their last respects. We then left for the cemetery and while they were transporting the casket to the gravesite, I walked with my aunt to see the other tombstones, including my grandfather's. I saw his photo on the stone and noticed he was a nice-looking man and I remember wondering, did I look like him? I later learned that he was a good man and worked very hard as a coal miner to support the family. He died from a lung infection most likely related to his work in the mines.

The service at the gravesite was starting and my grandmother was practically screaming as she cried. I didn't cry. I just held my mom tight. As they started to lower the casket into the grave, the priest threw holy water on it. I was told to throw a rose on the casket and I did. When the service was over, my cousin Kelly approached me and asked if she could write to me. My mom said it was okay, so I gave her my address.

I had a new family member from my father's side.

We started to walk away, and my mom was approached by her old friend Vera from Brazil who also lived on the East Coast. She told my mom that my grandmother told her she was not welcome at the funeral. Still angry from the day before, it was all she could handle. The next day, my mom made an appointment with a local doctor to give her a prescription for some tranquilizers. She got a few pills - just enough to help her get through the rest of the trip. We spent one more day at my aunt's house and then it was finally time to go home. I enjoyed the flight back since I knew we were going home. My Godfather picked us up at the airport, and I was happy to be there as was my mom. The trip brought back so many painful memories for her. I was glad it was over for both of us.

I got back into my routine going to school, doing homework, and being with my friends from the neighborhood. The diabetes never left, even though I wished I could have left it behind in New Jersey. I was lucky I made it through that ordeal without a serious high or low blood sugar event.

My cousin, Kelly wrote me a letter a few weeks after the funeral. She sent me her photo and told me life was getting hectic with her school. What did hectic mean? She was 16 and was more advanced with her vocabulary. She wanted me to write back to her, but for some reason I just wasn't interested. Besides, I didn't even know her and we were essentially strangers.

About a month later, my grandmother sent me a hundred dollars for my birthday which was still a few months away. Understandably my mom said, "Is this how she is going to make up for nine years of never seeing you and your father never contacting you? It's the least she could do." I told her I would really like a new bike with a banana seat on it. At the time, that was the new style for bikes and some of the kids in the neighborhood already had one. She told me I could spend it on whatever I wanted. Excited, I immediately went shopping with my Godfather to buy a bike. I chose a top-of-the-line pretty yellow and pink bike with a banana seat. We spent most of the money with some spare change. I was so happy and excited and couldn't wait to get it home. My Godfather assembled it and we left it in the basement until the weather got a little warmer. Once spring came, I was on that bike almost every day. Riding was good for my diabetes as it kept my blood sugar in line … or so I thought. I even gave kids from the neighborhood rides on it. The kids that were smaller than me would sit in back like a motorcycle and I would drive.

Fall arrived and it was time for my routine check-up. The nurse measured my height and weight as usual, and the doctor listened to my heart and checked my throat and neck. After he was done, he proceeded to tell my mom his findings. "She is doing well, however, I am suspicious in regards to her neck as there seems to be an enlargement on both sides." The doctor wanted a blood test to check for low thyroid and blood sugar level. My mom asked if this was serious and the doctor reassured her it was treatable. Another thing for my mom to worry about. In those days, the only way for a diabetic to check blood sugar was through a urine test with a test tube that was referred to as Clinitest. While I was no stranger to needles, I didn't know what a blood test was and as we waited that Saturday, I had a sick feeling in my stomach.

After waiting for almost an hour, the nurse called me to go back to a room. I wanted my mom there too. She sat me in a chair, and I put my left arm on the table. My heart started beating very fast and I felt cold. The nurse said, "hold steady - you will feel a little pinch." She proceeded to put the needle in my nine-year old vein, and it hurt. I remember watching my blood go into the tube. I was terrified, but I didn't move. It seemed like she took all of my blood, but then it was over and she untied the rubber band, took the needle out, and put a big cotton ball on my arm. She held it for a while then put a Band-Aid on it. My mom asked me if I was alright, and I told her I felt a little like throwing up. She thanked the nurse and we walked out and left the hospital. When we got into the car, my mom gave me my insulin injection and then she took me to McDonalds for breakfast. I ordered pancakes and sausage, which came with regular syrup. My mom told me I could only have a little bit of syrup but I really wanted the whole thing. I felt like I had been injured and I wanted the meal to console me. I wasn't allowed to finish all of the food.

The following Saturday I returned to the doctor. My mom was anxious about the results and prayed that it was nothing bad. The doctor started going over my results and proceeded to say that I tested low for thyroid and had hypothyroidism. He said that it was treatable by taking Synthroid every day in the morning and that we would have to keep an eye on the levels until we find out what medication strength works the best for me. He gave my mom the prescription and I remember being relieved that it wasn't another injection. The result of my blood sugar level was 300 mg/dl. That meant that my fasting blood sugar at the time of the test was very high since a normal range was 80 to 120 mg/dl. Despite this high number, my doctor felt this was a one-time number and didn't reflect my overall diabetes control. He was careful not to alarm my mom and I so that we would live our lives with as little stress as possible. He was always positive about my diabetes. He truly wanted me to grow up normally, without feeling like an outcast or thinking that diabetes was a barrier for me to accomplish anything and for that I owe him a great deal.

My mom filled my new prescription for the thyroid medication. I started to take it the next morning, on an empty stomach. After a month, they tested my thyroid level again and the doctor was impressed by the results. My neck was back to normal size and I had lost weight. This was a normal response to the medication and as a result, my metabolism was working correctly. We were very happy that this turned out well, and only required a pill, no shots! This was easy, and I only hoped I would stop needing the insulin injections. I had to monitor my thyroid levels from that point on, year after year. I was the first one in the family with a thyroid condition. Should I pat myself on the back? Did I win again? Although it was a nuisance to take a pill first thing in the morning, it was minor compared to the insulin injections.

Through a child's eyes, I thought it would be nice to fix the diabetes too. I remember the doctor telling me, "the cure for diabetes is just around the corner." That was over 40 years ago. How I wished he had been right. That encouragement gave me hope that there would be a cure soon, and I just stopped thinking about the diabetes for a while. Instead, I focused on school, friends, activities and my family. It was summer again and I was very active riding my bike around the neighborhood. I would take breaks, stopping in the house, opening the refrigerator and just grabbing what was staring at me to snack on. There was plenty of American cheese, and I ate several pieces. I didn't tell my mom, but I'm sure that prevented my blood sugar from bottoming out. I don't know how many times I saved myself from going into a severe hypoglycemic reaction. I knew God and his angels were with me. I had lost weight and I felt lighter so I really enjoyed being active outside playing hopscotch, jump rope, and going to the schoolyard. I never sat in the house. Being active helped me stay out of the hospital and keep my diabetes in control.

One weekend, we decided to go to the beach and have some fun swimming. My mom loved to soak up the sun and lay on the beach, and I loved the water. My mom would always ask if I needed to eat and most of the time, I wasn't hungry, but I ate a little something just so I could go back in the water. I would swim to the closest white buoy which was an accomplishment. I was so proud of myself that I learned how to swim and to float, and I was delighted that the sun was shining on me. There was nothing that could deter me from having my fun. These were days where there was no time to think about diabetes!

Summer was coming to a close and it was back to school. I started fifth grade and had a new teacher who, for the first time, was an older man. I didn't mind as long as he wasn't mean. It turned out he was quite strict and we clearly had to do what he said. He knew I was diabetic, as my mom always made that clear to all my teachers. A few weeks after school started, we had our first field trip. Our teacher was big into music so he scheduled a trip to Orchestra Hall in downtown Chicago. I had never seen any place like it. The only thing I knew about music is that I liked the Beatles. When we arrived,

I saw that the carpeting and the seats were very plush and red. The walls were ornate with carvings like a castle. I was a bit apprehensive, mostly because of my diabetes. I didn't want to drink juice there, and have other kids notice. I sat and listened as our teacher and the host started to tell the history of Orchestra Hall. We enjoyed the music while the orchestra played. Before I knew it, we had to go back on the bus and I felt good about having made it through without any major problems. It was an enjoyable field trip, something I had never experienced before.

Every week included a music day in our class. Little did I know that our teacher was having us rehearse for the next school Christmas show picking altos and sopranos. As we got closer to Christmas, the choices were narrowed to just a few who were going to be in the show. He planned a special performance of Silver Bells, and he selected three girls that he felt had the best voices for the song. The girls were Suzanne, Joy and myself. I was picked! I didn't know what to think or expect. Is this something I could do? We worked feverishly that final week before the show and had to stay after school to perfect our performance. This was my first real experience working in a team environment, and we depended on each other. We couldn't let Mr. Litner down or risk getting a bad grade.

The day of the Christmas show came and I knew Baba would come as the school was within walking distance for her. I was nervous, but I rehearsed my part hundreds of times it seemed, so I had to be ready. Suzanne, Joy and I wore the same outfits, red skirts and white tops since we were performing together.

The show began and we were the last ones to take the stage. The curtain opened and we were introduced. There was silence as our teacher got ready by the stage with his notes and wand. All eyes were on him. The music started and we began to sing. I couldn't see much since the lights were shining on us. It was better this way so I didn't have to see all those people looking at me. The group started to sing and then Suzanne, Joy and I performed our part of the song. I thought we sang fabulously, just like professionals. When the song was over, they turned down the lights and I looked around for Baba. I spotted her in the balcony and saw my mom was there too. She had left early from work to see me in the show and surprise me. I was so excited that they were both there to see me perform. It was one of the most joyful days of my life that I will never forget. My mom said I sang like an angel. I ran to see them in the audience and they both gave me a really big hug and kiss and said they loved to hear me sing and that they were so proud. This brought me closer to having more confidence in myself. I knew I had been selected because I could sing better than most of the kids in class. I was special and I felt it, and I did so well. However, I was glad it was over and the pressure was finally off. I could enjoy the Christmas break with my family and look forward to Christmas presents.

My teacher was truly one-of-kind and very inspirational. I learned a lot in his class, earned good grades and had a wonderful experience.

The school year passed quickly and spring arrived. I could barely wait for the warm weather and was already spending time outside. As always, I was walking to the playground armed with a little bag of sugar and a can of juice which is what my mom required for me to go there alone. As I was leaving the house, I ran into a girl who was also going to the playground. She said her name was Mary and she asked me what I was carrying. I said I was a diabetic and my mom made me take juice and sugar cubes with me in case I needed it. She proceeded to tell me she was a diabetic, too and sarcastically said her mom made her do that too, but that she did not have anything with her. I recall being surprised because I had never run into another diabetic before. I was certain I was the only living person on earth with diabetes, other than the ones in the Diabetes Forecast magazine. Mary was tall, thin and lanky and looked like she never ate anything. She had a long face. I had a round face. I felt obese next to her, even though I wasn't. We started to share stories about our diabetes, and I learned that I had been diagnosed far earlier than she had been. It could be why she was still so thin. We talked about chocolate chip cookies and how hard it was not to eat sugary treats. She hated the insulin injections too, but I didn't see any visible potholes on her skin like I had. I didn't know where Mary lived and she never invited me to her house. I only saw her once, although I knew she went to my school. I'm not sure if she liked me or not because we never pursued a friendship. My young mind wondered if she didn't want to know me because I reminded her of diabetes. Whatever the case, that was the only other child I knew with diabetes and she was also an only child. I ran home and told my mom I met Mary. She was glad I met someone else with diabetes and I shared how Mary's mom also told her to carry emergency sugar with her. I had finally met someone who dealt with this disease just like me. I wasn't the only one anymore. To this day, I often wonder how Mary is dealing with her diabetes or if she is still alive.

It was 1972 and things were changing in the two-flat home I lived in. My aunt, uncle and six and seven-year old cousins that lived upstairs were relocating to the suburbs. My uncle decided to build a house and move the family out of the city. It wasn't going to be a major move for my cousins because they were still young. Since the two-flat that we lived in was a shared expense, it was no longer affordable for us or my other uncles that were just out of college. My younger uncle Oleg was getting married soon and moving out, however, they were going to live in the city. We decided to look at some places in the suburbs and found a house that was built in 1964. It was still pretty new looking and the owners were relocating due to a job offer. Interestingly, the decision to buy that house was based on whether or not I approved when we saw it. I said the walls looked even so it was okay to move there. I really didn't think we would move. I thought looking at other people's homes was just something fun to do. Moving day came and everything was loaded on a rented truck. I never saw the only home I ever knew look so empty. I laid down on the carpeting in the living room and thought about all my experiences in the flat. When we had to leave I felt so sad. I was leaving all my friends, my school, the playground, the corner pharmacy where I bought my candy, the grocery store, the library, and the street where I took the city bus with Baba to go shopping. I was leaving my childhood memories behind.

I planned to keep in touch with a girl named Katy that I had known since second grade. I told her I was moving and she gave me her address so we could write. In the beginning, I wrote to her several times a month to let her know how I was doing and she did the same. Eventually, we started talking on the phone and that was helpful as I began to get used to my new surroundings. It was lonely having to move into the new house. Even though it had a back yard, I didn't spend much time there.

The first week after I moved in, there were two girls that lived across the street that came over and rang the doorbell. They introduced themselves as Arlene and Dina. It was a "welcome to the neighborhood" visit and they wanted to meet me and get to know me. I didn't tell them I was diabetic. We spent time together after school and sometimes went to each other's homes. I remember Arlene was a little more placid, and Dina was a bit boisterous. I took out my bike and rode it around, although it wasn't like the old neighborhood. The blocks were longer and the streets had more traffic. I was fortunate to meet Arlene and Dina before I started school, so at least I knew kids my own age. I wasn't going to be alone.

For the first six months I remember being intensely homesick. Though nice enough, these were not my childhood friends and the school was different. Instead of walking to school, I had to take a bus. Mom and Baba still made sure I had a lunch with me and extra juice just in case. At that time, the stores carried small cans of Hawaiian Punch and I would either have a can in my lunch bag or in my purse. The move caused me to become more introverted. I was very tense about starting a new school and not having any close friends, plus I was diabetic and had to deal with that, too. I continued to wear the pendant necklace under my clothes that indicated that I had diabetes. Again, I so wanted to fit in and be like the other kids.

The first day of school in a strange place was intimidating. I walked to the bus on the first day with my next-door neighbor boy named Danny. My mom had talked to Danny's mom and asked if he could walk me to the bus stop so I wouldn't be alone for the first month or so. Danny wasn't too keen on the idea, but he did it anyway. He didn't say too much to me, maybe grunted "hello", and then proceeded to walk in front of me to the bus stop. I had the impression he didn't like me much, or having to walk with me to the bus stop like I was his girlfriend. I carried heavy schoolbooks, my lunch bag, as well as my purse with extra juice in it. Once we got to the bus stop, he would meet up with some friends and they totally ignored me. I felt like I didn't really have anyone to talk to, and that was hard for me.

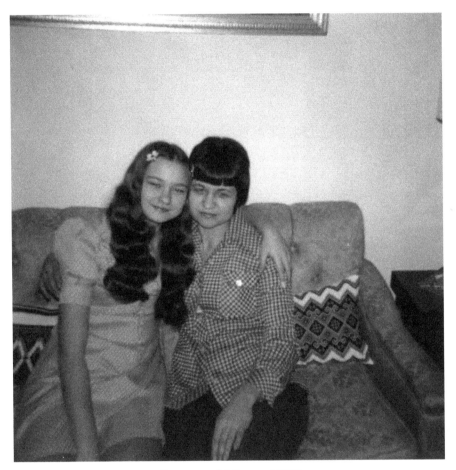

Lucy and Mama 1975

I started sixth grade at the junior high which was much different than grade school. This was larger with more hallways and classrooms and a huge cafeteria. We had a one hour lunch break and I had to get used to eating a sandwich instead of a warm meal Baba would prepare at the old house when I would come home for lunch.

We had homeroom where we started each day with a dedicated teacher. It was really nice not having to be introduced as new. Everyone who started sixth grade was a new student! The only difference was nobody knew me because I wasn't from around the area. On the first day, I sat next to a girl named Janey who had blue eyes and blonde hair. She looked a bit like me, only a little thinner. She really wanted to get to know me and kept asking me lots of questions. I liked her because she was the first friendly face I met since I moved to the area. I remember she had an odd odor that I could not figure out but I was still friendly to her. Who was I to judge? I had diabetes.

The same week, another girl named Lila approached me in the hallway and asked me if I liked Janey. I told her I thought she was nice. Lila told me nobody liked Janey and that I shouldn't hang around with her. She didn't give me a reason why, just that nobody really liked her. Was it because of her strange odor? I never really knew why, but after Lila told me that I started to distance myself from Janey. I wanted the other kids to like me and if I liked Janey, they might look down on me and maybe talk about me, too. God forbid I be different. Having Diabetes was different enough. Who else had to get injections, never eat sugar and faint unexpectedly? I felt really bad distancing myself from Janey because I knew what she was going through. I saw the other kids in the school as typical spoiled suburban kids. I started to hear swear words in the hallway as I passed by lockers. They would hurry to get to class before the bell rang and it was like Grand Central Station. When school was over, we had to make sure we got on the right bus to get home. There were rowdy boys at the back of the bus that created commotion every day. It was never peaceful.

After a few days at this school, I became edgy and panicky. I missed home, I wanted my mom, and I felt sick to my stomach. This happened for a long time after I started school there. I had to go the school nurse several times, and each time they would call my mom to come and pick me up and take me home. After I got home, I was relieved. I was with Baba. My mom would call Baba and ask how I was, and she said I felt better when I got home. My mom was at her wits end after a while and finally talked to a school counselor, Mr. Robitini. We called him Rob for short. They talked to him and told me that if I was feeling this way again, I should go talk with Rob unless I was really dying, and then I could go home. I was scared of Rob. He was loud, big, overweight, bald and had a beard. He could have been a pirate for all I knew. I wasn't the invincible kid that came from the city anymore. Instead, I had become very shy and insecure. This environment was hard for me to deal with. I always had diabetes on my mind and the possibility of low blood sugar. I didn't want to faint and have the kids find out. Consequently, I became less physically active. I would go to school, go home, watch TV and do homework. We did have physical education in school, but it wasn't anywhere near the level of activity I had when we lived in the city. Now if I had the nervous sick-to-my-stomach feeling at school, I had to go to Rob's office. There was no way to go home unless I was *actually* ill. Rob did his best to comfort me and I would just sit and listen. I can't remember our conversations, but eventually the feelings started to subside and I got used to the environment. I had to calm myself down, what else could I do? As long as no one knew I was diabetic, I was okay.

I had started some new classes including science and art. I really liked both subjects and they didn't bore me like math or English. I lost myself in art and drawing would help me forget about other things. I hated when the class was over because I just wanted to keep drawing, painting and creating. The art teacher really enjoyed my work and said I was very good. I forgot all about diabetes when I was in that class and always looked forward to it. I finally started to make friends that I saw more often in the same classes. There was a really shy girl named Beth that shared a locker next to me, and I would say "hi" to her and start talking. She had long hair like me and I complimented her. I found out that we lived close to each other in the same neighborhood. She also liked art, doing crafts and reading teen magazines. We exchanged phone numbers and kept in touch, even when school was out.

I don't remember having low blood sugar too many times after I started attending the new school, although I frequently felt sick to my stomach. A few months after I began talking to Rob, I remember raising my hand to be excused from music class. All the kids looked at me as I left the classroom. I went to the nurse and she checked my urine sugar level. It wasn't too high and she told me I could go back to class. I was relieved that no one said anything when I came back to class 10 minutes later. I thought it was a non-event. After class, Beth shared that the teacher told the whole class that I had diabetes and not to make any comments or make fun of me when I came back. She explained that I had to go to the nurse sometimes to check my sugar level. I felt so uneasy and I wanted to cry. Why did the teacher tell the whole world I was diabetic? I felt so low, how could I face everyone now? Now that they knew I had a disease, I was sure they were going to talk about me behind my back and make fun of me. I was screaming inside but I couldn't do anything, the damage was done. After that I felt like the whole school knew my secret. How was I going to fit in and who would want to be friends with me? I'm different; I have a medical condition. I have to get shots every day. Who does that? They can eat sugary cereals for breakfast, have cake and donuts and never blink an eye. Beth continued to be my friend, and never said anything bad about the diabetes. She was self-conscious about having a large nose, and always talked about it. I never had an issue with it, but she did.

The next day in school I felt like all the kids were talking about me. I tried to hide when walking in the hallways by not looking at anyone. It might have been just my imagination, but it felt real. There's the diabetic (ha-ha.) She has to check her urine (ha-ha.) Why did we move to this town? I was perfectly fine in the other neighborhood. I buried myself in my studies and for the most part stayed out of everyone's way. I tried to get good grades, and I usually did well except for math.

In the meantime, my blood sugars were always high. I would try to wake up to go to school and my mom couldn't pull me out of my bed because I was so tired. I wasn't watching anything that I ate. My stomach would grumble at night to the point it woke me. Once, I actually got up to eat an apple strudel that Baba bought and kept hidden away in the pantry. At school I sometimes felt like a walking zombie, going from class to class. My family thought I just didn't want to go to school, but I was so exhausted from my poor diet and it was difficult to get up. In the morning when I had class, I couldn't focus and pay attention. I had to get caught up after school when I did the homework. I had my uncle help me with math sometimes because it was my worst subject.

Mom finally took me to the doctor and we had to increase the insulin by several units until I reached 100. That was the number that worked. I think that the stress levels at school added to my sugar level and it was like a yo-yo. When my adrenaline went up, it directly affected my blood sugar level. Adrenaline acts like sugar in the body and for a diabetic that's not good. There is no insulin to compensate for higher blood sugar, and no way to measure it. It was adding insult to injury. In a diabetic, higher blood sugar levels make one crave more sugar and create a false feeling like you are starving. I didn't have an understanding of this process and so I just kept eating things I shouldn't have. Since my mom was always at work and Baba used to love to bake, I would just help myself. I had not learned about hidden sugars in many foods including things like ketchup. I was eating unknown amounts of sugar all the time.

It was a difficult time in my diabetic life. All of the changes including my school, my environment, trying to make new friends and fit in combined with becoming less active was taking its toll. This was the first time I was experiencing real stress in my life and it was affecting my diabetes. As a result, I was moodier because the high blood sugar made me lethargic. I didn't know that the combination of poor diet and reduced activity would have such an overpowering effect on me. I never really complained, I just went along with it and still tried to pretend I wasn't a diabetic because I didn't want to be. This was a new school and they weren't supposed to find out that I was different. I still wanted so badly to be "normal". Poor management of my diabetes felt like I was taking drugs. I felt tired – almost high, and didn't really care about anything.

At school I tried to make new friends, but I had become so shy that it was difficult. I went to my classes and if someone was interested in talking with me, I would typically respond, but otherwise I was generally like a wall flower, trying to stay out of sight and everyone's way. The way I viewed my peers included the "normal" ones, the cheerleaders that I didn't talk to, the instigators always trying to make trouble, the drama kids who liked to be seen, the "cool" kids (some of whom smoked or did drugs), and the studious types who kept to themselves. I was shy and stayed really close to my family. I felt they were the only ones I could trust in this new environment.

One winter day Dina and Arlene came over to my house after school and asked me to go with them to see a friend they knew. I tagged along and felt like the third wheel. We arrived at their friend's house and a red - haired, stocky girl came out in hip-hugger pants and a school letter jacket. They talked and joked briefly and then the girl said she had some marijuana. She pulled out a plastic bag containing what appeared to be mini cigarettes.

Arlene and especially Dina seemed interested and they asked me if I wanted some. I knew these were drugs. In homeroom one day, the teacher burned something that smelled like marijuana so we would know what to look out for and understand that it was dangerous. I recognized the smell right away when the red-haired girl lit it. Even if it had been regular cigarettes, I had no desire to smoke it. I became fearful and my hands turned cold. Did they expect me to smoke it? As she offered me some, I said, "Oh it's getting late and my mom should be home soon, so I have to go." I quickly pulled myself out of that jam and then just walked home without Dina and Arlene. I think I was startled at that moment more than anything else and I was also hoping they wouldn't come after me or think I would tattle on them. After I turned the corner (out of sight) I started to run home. I looked around me to see if they were following me, but I was safe.

My 12-year-old mind was thinking I already have to give injections to myself every day, something I didn't want to do, and then these girls want to take drugs? From that moment on, my whole perspective changed on people who intentionally did non-prescription drugs. I would do anything to be drug-free, to be completely healthy, and these girls wanted to intentionally harm themselves. I remember back in the city seeing some protestors from the 1960's, men with long unkempt hair and beards and scantily dressed women walking around looking like they were on drugs. I saw them as agitators. I didn't want to be in that group and my mind went to that memory when the red-haired girl pulled the marijuana from her pocket. I don't want to harm myself, I thought. I've been through so much already with the diabetes and I was still very young. I suddenly felt alone again, and that I didn't fit in. I didn't really care to hang around with those girls; we had nothing in common.

The girls in school all started talking about wearing a bra. I didn't have anything to fill a bra, but they wanted to show that they were going to be teenagers ahead of their time. I didn't think anything of it and I wondered why they would bother. I came home and told my mom that the girls were talking about bras and she laughed and said, "you don't need a bra." A few weeks went by and the girls were checking who was wearing bras. One of the girls came up behind my back and pulled on my shirt to see if something would make a snapping sound. I was sure they were going to pick on me. I was now living in suburbia and I felt there were standards I needed to keep up with. I believed the suburban girls kept up with everything. They didn't hear my bra snap because I was wearing an undershirt. I felt embarrassed and I didn't move - I just waited until they left. I didn't flinch or say anything. I kept my cool but wanted to cry.

I came home and told my mom the story. I'd told her I had better get a bra or I will be the oddball and they won't leave me alone. My mom agreed only because she didn't want them to bother me about it. I went shopping that weekend because I couldn't wait any longer. I started to try on different bras in the store to figure out what size would fit. It felt like I was wearing a big rubber band across my chest. Why were the girls at school promoting this? It was downright uncomfortable and seemed to restrict my breathing. But I didn't say anything, I just pretended I was happy and we left the store.

I *had* to fit in and if this is what it took, this was easy. Diabetes was the hard part. I got through the first day of school wearing the bra. When I got home, I immediately took it off and put on my comfortable undershirt. What an ordeal. To be honest, I think the injections were less of a problem than that first bra! About a week went by and I wore the bra to school every day. A bunch of girls quickly ran by in back of me and one of them snapped my bra. As they left, I'd had a smile on my face. Ha, I'm covered! They can't say I don't fit in anymore. It felt good not to be different for a moment, although I knew that was temporary.

Every day at school we had to participate in gym class and all the girls had to wear the same gym suit. It was a stretchy burgundy one-piece with a zipper in the front. I hated it. When I initially tried it on, I noticed my butt stuck out. My mom would give me injections on both sides of my butt and I had developed hypertrophy which is a mound that forms when injections are given in the same spot all the time. It looks like a deformity, and it doesn't really go away. I would notice it in the mirror when I put on my gym suit in the locker room and I was really self-conscious about it. The only thing that was good about that class was the gym teacher who was very nice and pleasant. We would leave our gym suits in the lockers for the next day. One day I noticed someone was switching my suit with another, and it was a different size. I complained to the gym teacher and then told my mom. They immediately got me another suit and my mom sewed my name (by hand) in black letters on the front of the suit. I thought the problem was solved. Who would want to take my gym suit now that it had my name on it? Three days later, I came to class and noticed someone had cut the thread on my

A DIABETIC'S JOURNEY

name and it was damaged. I was very upset. Who was doing this to me? I took it home and my mom fixed it. From that point, I took my suit home every day - I didn't know who my enemy was.

I didn't pay attention to my blood sugar much when I started junior high. Thank God I didn't have to prick my finger during those years to keep checking it. I already wasn't sure if I would make it through junior high in this environment. I constantly felt tired and I didn't have any low blood sugar. I kept saying to myself, "I don't have diabetes, I'm just like any one of the kids, I'm normal!" I went along with the curriculum, kept more to myself and didn't want anyone to bother me too much, unless they seemed nice.

Even in junior high, my mom still wanted me to attend Ukrainian school every Saturday to learn about my heritage and history. I hated missing the cartoons on TV, but I had a full schedule. I had homework during the week for both schools. Ukrainian school was on Saturday from 9 a.m. to 2 p.m. so my only day off was Sunday. I had made some friends in junior high, and I also had my Ukrainian friends.

At another visit to my doctor he said I was doing fine, and continued monitoring my thyroid and adjusting my insulin. Hormones affect blood sugar levels and as I entered puberty mine were changing. I had no idea how to compensate for this new reality. Balancing carbohydrates, fat, proteins, insulin and now hormones. What a task! I could always lean on my mom with all these issues which made me feel a little more secure. She told me she began menstruating when she was 14. It didn't seem fair that I started my period younger. Then she told me how hard it was when hers started to get any feminine hygiene products. As far as that goes, I guess I was luckier.

Beginning to get my period along with diabetes made my blood sugars go out of whack. It seemed like every month I would experience high blood sugar around that time. As a result, I craved sweets. This had become a convenient excuse for me not to avoid them. My body was changing and I didn't know how to compensate except to eat sweets – candy, baked goods, ice cream, whatever satisfied me at the time and I enjoyed eating those things immensely. This in turn would make me tired and yet, I had no idea why I felt that way. Another byproduct of uncontrolled diabetes *and* puberty was frequent yeast infections that I began to think was normal around my period. I had great discomfort and the high sugar intake was fueling the yeast and causing terrible itching. I was too embarrassed to ask any other girls or my mom about why it was happening.

Although I had cheated throughout childhood by eating sweets, it didn't affect me as much because I was so active. I continued to miss all my friends in the old neighborhood. I felt like things had gotten more difficult for me since we made the move to the suburbs. I was getting used to junior high, however I had become moodier than ever. Most of the time I felt out of sorts where I just didn't want anyone to bother me. My sugars were up and the hormones were firing. Not a good combination. This was a miserable time and my mom had no idea how I'd been feeling. I tried to get good grades in school, and I passed my classes without a lot of studying. Looking back, I'm not completely sure how I did it. Despite all of the adjustments I had made, school became routine. I didn't want to disappoint my mom and wanted her to be proud of me.

Soon I started to fill out and needed to update my bra wardrobe. I also needed new clothes, but it was difficult as we couldn't afford too much. My mom went back to high school and then enrolled in classes for keypunch operating to try and earn more money. She was now working in an office and not in a factory. Her change in occupation meant we were able to buy some clothes, but I certainly didn't have as much as the other kids in school. Most of them came from a two-parent household. My mom wanted me to have things the other kids had. It was painful for her that we didn't have my father to take care of us. The medication I needed was not cheap and I needed insulin injections every day. We did not have health insurance when she worked in the factory. Eventually, my mom landed a job that offered health insurance for employees and their families. Insurance covered 80 percent of my medications which was a relief for our budget.

One day I started crying because I had a tremendous amount of pain in my lower abdomen on the left side. I was bent over and could not function. After seeing the doctor, he admitted me to the hospital. The hospital did a series of tests to rule out anything serious. My mom came to visit me in the hospital and asked what was happening and I remember them talking in the hallway so that I would not hear. The next day, the nurse came in and said "You have your period, when was the last time you had it?" I shrugged my shoulders like a typical 12-year old would. I didn't know how to answer because I didn't keep track. The next day the doctor released me from the hospital. They never determined why I had so much pain. Life eventually went back to my version of normal, whatever that was.

The school year was almost over and I would have my first summer in the new house and finally become a teenager having turned 13. When school ended, I got bored and lonely. My mom was at work during the day and I was with Baba. I didn't have any real close friends and I stayed in most of the time. I tried to ride my bike but I didn't have the energy like I did when we lived in the city. I kept myself busy by doing different crafts. My mom had bought me enough yarn to make a blanket, my first real project. Baba liked to do embroidery, and I liked to crochet. When she was working on something, I would work on my blanket. I was sitting most of the time and not really into doing anything active. Baba liked to make sweet lemonade and I loved having it. Baba also liked to garden. Every day in the summertime she would tend to her tomatoes, cucumbers, lettuce, carrots, dill, and zucchini. We had wonderful fresh salads and vegetables every summer. I loved that I could finally relax and not have to rush to go to school, although I didn't have much energy. I really looked forward to the weekends when I could do something with my mom.

When I wasn't crocheting, I was working on a paint by number kit that my mom had bought. I enjoyed doing it because I felt like I accomplished something and it made me forget about my health problems. I would get so engrossed, Baba had to tear me away from painting so I could eat lunch. All I wanted to do was paint. I would lose myself in the project. I wasn't bored anymore, and when I wasn't in the mood to paint, I would watch TV. The summer went by too fast … and just as I was getting used to it.

Fall arrived and I religiously watched the Partridge Family every week. I never missed an episode. David Cassidy was so cute he made me forget about everything. I would read all about him in the teen magazines that my mom would buy for me. I had all the 45s of the Partridge Family songs and played them for hours in my room. My cousin would come over sometimes and we would record ourselves singing to their songs. It was an obsession and it made me feel like a normal teenage girl.

I started school again and this was my final year of junior high. I had made it through the first year, I couldn't believe it. It was the mid-1970s and everything was changing including fashion and music. My mom made a lot of my clothes and I had a certain top with puffy sleeves that I tied in the back. I wore it to school and there would always be someone who tried to untie it all the time when I wasn't looking. I never knew who did those things to me. I started to accept that I would continue to be picked on because it started when I arrived there.

That year I tried to make friends with some girls in the school courtyard during break. They were all sitting in a group on the sidewalk by the school entrance and I joined them. I was still shy and didn't know what to say. One girl had brought Avon perfume and we all smelled the bottle and sprayed some on. I decided I would complement the perfume, ask their names and start talking about it. I thought that girl was so lucky to have the perfume; it smelled so nice. Nobody paid attention to what I had to say, so I just sat there and listened to them talk. They talked about David Cassidy and boys in the class. I started to pay more attention to who they had crushes on and then I made my own observations. These girls were more conservative so I stuck with them. They were studious and got good grades.

This particular year they started a new class called Home Economics. We were taught cooking, sewing, and different craft projects. I didn't know what to expect, but I gave it my best. The first thing that the teacher showed us was how to cook. I thought it would be boring. This was something Baba did and I didn't think it was glamorous. Well, the first thing we made was blueberry muffins! Hey, I thought, this class might not be half bad! I learned how to mix and bake and yes, I did eat. I forgot about the diabetes again for a second and enjoyed myself. I also wanted to fit in and not make a big deal about not being able to eat sugar. The teacher had us buy a recipe box so we could write down the recipes on 3x5 index cards and keep them. The muffins were the first thing I made at home and showed everyone I could make something different to eat. I thought they were delicious and so I continued making them for a long time.

In class, we would rotate doing the cleanup of the dishes after preparing food. I did the dishes the first time and did not wear plastic gloves. One of the girls made a comment that I should do the dishes with gloves on. She even told the teacher. I didn't see what the big deal was, but she had said her mom always did the dishes with gloves on and that was the proper way to do it. My mom had to buy me gloves for washing dishes in class. I couldn't believe it. The next time I went to class and when it was my turn to do dishes, I wore those gloves. It was so difficult to use them as the dishes kept sliding out of my hands and I would drop them sometimes. The same girl saw what happened and she kept making derogatory comments to me. She kept bossing me around and I finally got fed up and started yelling at her to stop picking on me. I told her that she should do the dishes and that she always gets away without doing them. I was very upset. The teacher stepped in and I told her what happened. The teacher tried not to take sides, but she saw how upset I was. Then the girl started whispering about me, like I was a bad person, but it didn't matter because I stood up for myself. This was the first time I did that and it felt good. After that, I tried to stay away from her.

The next thing we did in that class was sewing and I liked doing crafts. It also meant I didn't have to interact too much with the other girls and I showed them that I was very good in doing my work. The teacher didn't even help me that much, but a lot of the other girls needed help. I had always watched my mom sew at home so I was more familiar with it. One day, the teacher said we needed to choose a project. I decided to make a southern colonial flag because I really enjoyed this part of American history. My mom got me all the material and helped me to cut the pieces at home. When I finally finished, I remember being very proud that I had tackled such a large project.

In addition to that class, I had also started a new art class. This brought out more creativity as I learned how to draw, use watercolors, and mixed media. This was another class I looked forward to and I even had a drawing portfolio book. I was very good in drawing and the art teacher was always pleased with my work. I don't think any of the students hated that class. We were all so diligent and paid attention to our work. The teacher told us to draw something from a picture, so I decided to draw a watercolor of my house. It turned out very well and I still have it to this day. I was very proud of it and the teacher gave me an A.

Like most girls, I dreaded gym class when I had my period. It was the most miserable time in my young life for exercising. I never knew how I was going to feel or what we would do in gym class every day. Sometimes we would do something simple like badminton, and other times we would have to run or dance. The latter was the worst. At least with the badminton I could fake it and just stand and pretend I was moving to get the birdie. When it came to moving around more I would do as little as possible when the teacher wasn't watching. I never complained to anyone. I would just suffer quietly.

I did well in school that year, averaging a B plus with a few A's. My only problem was math, but somehow, I made it through that too. My mom was proud of me and didn't expect anything less than good grades. She wanted me to succeed, and so did Baba. Baba never had a formal education and so she wanted her children and grandchildren to graduate. The importance of education was instilled in me at a young age. I was not aware that my family ever treated me as though I had a medical condition. To them, I was normal and could do anything other kids did. I had to take medication and watch my sugar intake, but they never talked about what could happen to me because I had diabetes. They didn't want me to worry. All I wanted to do was fit in.

The next school year came with new classes and getting to know new students. I met a girl named Deb that acted like she was in her 40's. She used to call me "kid" in a way I enjoyed. Nobody had given me a nickname before. We became friends and I remember learning so many things from her. She was a "latch-key" kid because her parents worked and she had to be independent. We would hang around in between classes and I could count on her if I didn't understand something. Finally, I had a close friend at school. She acted very adult-like and I admired that about her. She was not shy, like me. She knew some boys and when around them, acted more like she belonged in high school than in junior high. She had short hair, wore lipstick, cologne, eyeshadow and mascara. She had what I didn't have … no fear. I studied how she acted so I could gain confidence. I liked hanging around with her because she was easy going, but she smoked cigarettes which bothered me. She used to sneak in the bathroom to smoke and I could only put up with it for so long. Eventually, I realized she was not my speed and the friendship fell apart.

I started being friendlier with Beth whose locker was next to mine. She was shy, had long hair like me and we would talk about our classes and the other kids at school. She knew I had diabetes and it didn't make any difference to her. I believe she understood shyness, and was even more introverted than I. Beth was the first real friend I had since I moved into the new neighborhood. We became very good friends.

All through junior high, I never had low blood sugar. I'm not sure if it was because of my poor diet or not exercising, but I suspect I was just barely getting away with high blood sugar. A lot of the time I just wasn't hungry for healthy food. Nobody knew what I ate during the night. I continued to have a hard time getting up in the morning. My blood sugar was high and that made me very tired. I would finally start to recover during class after 10:00 a.m. when my insulin would kick in.

Beth would call me on the phone sometimes and that felt great. Someone actually wanted to talk to me. We would get together at each other's homes and just spend time. She loved watching David Cassidy's show and listening to the Partridge Family, too. There were other girls I knew at school, but they were just acquaintances – I would say "hello" when I saw them in the halls or at lunch.

We had our first school field trip out of state to visit a famous zoo in Wisconsin. I tried not to get nervous about it, but in the back of my mind I always had to remember my diabetes was going with me. I made sure I ate well and brought juice and snacks in case I needed it. There was going to be a lot of walking around, it was a much bigger zoo than the ones where I lived. I didn't bring insulin with me because I was only getting one injection a day and didn't think I would need anymore. The doctor never mentioned that I would need to adjust anything in case it went high.

I took a camera with me and when we got there it felt like I was on another planet. The zoo was enormous and I didn't want to get lost. I made sure I stayed closed to everyone. Every time I saw an animal, I took a picture. It felt so great! I was actually enjoying the trip, even though there was a lot of walking to do. Sometimes I had to run to catch up with the other kids who were walking fast. I certainly didn't want to stray away from the crowd. I tried not to be nervous and fit in. I always felt like I was bringing up the rear and following everybody. Most everyone was walking with a buddy except me. I just kept taking pictures and before I knew it, it was 1:00 p.m. and we had to get back on the bus to go home. In a way, I was relieved. Most of the kids were having such a great time, they didn't want to go back. I got on the bus with my camera and overloaded purse. I was proud that I had a camera and could take my own pictures. I couldn't wait to get them developed to show everyone. We ate our lunches on the bus going back.

When I got home, I gave the film to my mom so she could take me to drop it off at the local Fotomat the next day. Fotomat was like a stand-alone phone booth and film could be dropped off like a drive-thru. I wanted to experience that because it was unusual and fun. When I dropped it off, the attendant said it would be ready in a few days. All I could think about was how the photos would turn out. I was very careful to take pictures that were centered and I didn't shake the camera. I learned from my uncle who taught me how to take photographs.

After a few days, we picked up the pictures. My mom paid for them and I grabbed them out of her hand. My mom was still standing at the booth and I rushed to open the envelope. The pictures of the animals at the zoo came out, but there was a big brown splattered line running through them that interfered with the picture, actually blocking the image in some of them. I showed my mom and said, "look, these are ruined!" The attendant apologized and said they were having a problem with the development of some films and it appeared mine happened to be one of them. I was so upset and angry, I wanted to cry. The pictures I took were nice, but they were ruined by their processing. These were my first real memories on film from my school trip and now I didn't have anything. All the attendant could do was give us a brand new roll of film. It was one of the most awful days of my young life!

I still felt like almost nothing went very well after I moved. It seemed that I had to try twice as hard to get something to go right. Whenever I experienced another disappointment, I thought about what sweet thing I could eat. I wanted something forbidden that I could indulge in and feel better, at least for a minute or so until my blood sugar went up. I would ask my mom if she could take me to Burger King which was my favorite restaurant, so I could get some French fries. Then I would have a small ice cream cone. My mom typically felt sorry for me, and sometimes she gave in just in an attempt to make me feel better. I would simply adjust my insulin later if the blood sugar went too high. Too much fat and sugar are the worst things for a diabetic. First the sugar goes up, and then goes up even higher when the fat goes through the body several hours later - even into the next day, unless exercise follows. In my case I didn't exercise much anymore, so my blood sugar was often elevated. I continued to try my best in regular school, Ukrainian school on Saturdays and with my diabetes. It was all so stressful, but I somehow managed to get out of bed every morning on time to take my insulin injections, thyroid pill, eat breakfast and then get on the bus. That was my routine and there was no changing it. I could not skip my medications and I always had to have breakfast. If I didn't eat all of it, or only ate part of it, I could have serious problems later in the morning. I continued to want to have a sweet roll in the morning like the rest of the family, but all I could do was watch. I would have my single piece of toast, a scrambled egg and some orange juice. I wasn't permitted to have any sugary cereal, only Cherrios with milk which tasted like cardboard to me. My breakfast was so boring I couldn't stand it! All the kids were always bragging about eating Pop-Tarts. I was only imagining the indulgence. I felt deprived and it was getting worse as I got older. Willpower is a struggle for anyone, but for a child it was even more difficult. I struggled and I struggled.

There were vending machines at school and sometimes I would absolutely crave barbecued potato chips. When nobody was looking, I would buy them and then sneak them in a room somewhere and eat them. I could have eaten 20 bags.

At home I would look at myself (front and back in my underwear) in the dresser mirror and noticed that I was developing cellulite on my thighs. I didn't like it. Most of the girls in school were very skinny and didn't have this problem. I couldn't understand why this was happening to me. Cellulite should only happen to older people, not a 13-year old. I watched all the girl gymnasts on television during the Olympics and even they didn't have those kind of thighs. All I could do is sigh. This was another problem in my eyes – one I could actually see. There was hypertrophy on my butt from the frequent injections. I always wanted to wear long shirts so they would cover everything. At this age, I always wanted to look as well as I possibly could. I was fearful about anyone pointing out my flaws because there was really nothing I could do about it, and junior high was the worst place to stand out. I felt that the kids in my school were rude.

The school year was going by fast and soon it would be spring. I could not wait for this year to be over and finally leave this school behind. I seemed to face non-stop challenges from the first minute I stepped in the door and it seemed the good memories were far and few between.

May of 1975 was just around the corner and it was time to get ready for graduation. I made it! I made it through the adjustments, the difficulties, my illnesses, the studies and survived the classmates who were not kind. As a teenager I didn't feel it could be any worse than this particular season of my life. I was grateful for my family – they meant everything to me. Mom, Baba and my uncles were my protectors, my shock absorbers so to speak. Without them, I'm not sure how I could have made it through.

As part of the baby-boomer generation, my graduating class had more than 800 students. We had rehearsals in the gym the week before graduation so that we knew how to walk and where to go. I had to keep in mind that the building was hot, although the ceremony would be in the evening. Graduation day rolled around and I was tense. I was hoping I wouldn't fall on stage or do something stupid. We were not required to wear graduation robes and my mom had bought me a beautiful dress that was navy-colored, floor-length, long-sleeved with orange and white flowers and a white collar. I felt like a princess and I remember fitting right in with all the other girls.

My mom and Baba came to my graduation along with my uncles. As we started to walk in, some parents would yell their child's name and wave. They were happy to see them graduating. It was my turn to walk and I found myself looking towards the floor and trying not to turn red from embarrassment. My blood sugar was likely high from the excitement. I loved my dress and felt really good wearing it. I think it saved me. I made it to my chair with great relief.

My name came up and I had to walk by myself up to the stage with all eyes on me. I carefully held my gown so I wouldn't trip on the stairs. I walked up a few stairs, got on stage and shook the principal's hand and received my diploma. I had a diploma and I felt proud. It felt really good to graduate. My anxiety was diminishing, I felt like I could breathe again. I scurried through the crowd looking for mom and Baba and my uncles. My mom found me and I showed her my diploma. She gave me a big hug and kiss, so did Baba. They were so proud of me. Even Mr. Robotini, my school counselor, put his arm around my shoulders and gave me a hug. He was glad to see I'd survived all the difficulties when I first came to the school. He was my first real adult friend. We talked for a short while and then left to go home.

I felt just a bit sad that I was leaving my school, only because I felt it marked my transition out of childhood into a new phase. I definitely wouldn't miss some of the difficult memories tied to our move from the city though.

I was happy the summer was just around the corner and I planned to spend more time outside. My cousins lived about five miles away and I looked forward to seeing them and their adorable new baby more often. My uncle would drop off his little baby girl at my house so Baba could babysit her newest granddaughter. When I was at their house, his wife would always talk up a storm. She knew everyone from church and loved to gossip. At one point she had the nerve to mention that she thought I had "sick blood". This really offended my mom and she quickly came to my defense. Both my mom and I took that comment very badly and talked bad about her when we got in the car. How could she do that to me? We were family! I felt very small. I started to think that they were spreading rumors that I had "sick blood". I wanted to cry, but I was angry at the same time. Why am I stuck with this diabetes when I never asked for it? I just wanted to be normal.

After we got home, I was still thinking about that comment. I eventually brushed it off and continued to enjoy my summer. My uncle Alex took his kids to summer camp and I wasn't going anywhere. I stayed at home most of the time, did some cartwheels in the backyard, watched TV and worked on some crafts to keep me busy. Mom was at work and Baba was always making something to eat and doing the housework. Baba would really make some wonderful desserts. She would always use yeast in her baking, and the things she made were so delicious, I couldn't help but eat them when they were fresh. She would make pyrohy, right out of the oven, and a sheet coffee cake with plums inside. I remember I would have several pieces of the coffee cake and Baba never stopped me, she wanted me to enjoy it. I tried not to overdo it because the diabetes police was always sitting on my shoulder telling me, not too much, not too much, but, I was getting away with it. Nobody knew, but my body sure did. It was taking a toll on my health. No matter how I tried to sneak things into my mouth, there was no fooling my body. I felt lethargic and sad and then I would think about every kid my age who was not diabetic and how they were enjoying their summer.

That summer, I spent more time outdoors in the backyard with Baba in her garden and we would sit and talk with the next-door neighbor, Mrs. Burnett. I remember she had a little dog that never left her lap. Mrs. Burnett was closer to Baba's age and she spoke Polish, so Baba was able to understand her, even though she spoke Ukrainian. I would get some sun sitting outside, and just listen to them talk. One day I developed a small round white spot on my shoulder. I covered it with makeup. This was the start of what turned out to be vitiligo later on in my life.

My birthday came around and I turned 14. We would always go to the fabric stores to look at the newest fashions and I was happy that my mom could sew clothes for me. She made me a cute yellow top with puffy sleeves and on the front of it Baba embroidered a beautiful butterfly. I was so excited to wear it. It was original, and everyone commented on how nice it was. It was the 1970's. I had long hair almost to my waist and wanted to wear the latest styles. Fashion got my mind off of food and gave me something else to enjoy.

My oldest cousin in New Jersey was getting married for the first time. She had asked me if I would be one of her bridesmaids and told me she had already picked out the dresses. They were long peach-colored polyester dresses with matching artificial flower headpieces. My cousin had shipped the dress to me and it fit nicely. I was concerned about who I would be standing up with, and my cousin told me it was a relative of her fiancé, about 3 years older than I. In a few weeks we would drive 17 hours to the East Coast for the wedding. All the relatives on my mom's side were there along with close family friends. We would be seeing people we hadn't seen for years. My mom even splurged and bought a dress for herself instead of sewing one.

The drive to my aunt's house was very long and we made several stops along the way. My mom packed breakfast for me along with my medications and then gave me my injection later that morning. My aunt and uncle and cousins greeted us. Soon thereafter we settled into our beds and just crashed from fatigue. It was just so nice to sleep after the long trip. The following day, I went to the wedding rehearsal. I was the junior bridesmaid, the youngest one standing up in the wedding. My aunt loved to cook and always made a hearty breakfast. I made sure I had enough to eat, because I didn't want to have a fainting episode. My mom was there too, so I felt more comfortable. I met my cousin's fiancé for the first time. I wasn't too impressed, he had a poof hairdo and a beard and mustache. Still, I was happy for my cousin.

I met the young man I was standing up with and I took a double take. He had long blonde hair past his shoulders, and he looked to be about 17 years old. I was immediately taken aback by his hair as it was almost as long as mine. He didn't talk much and I wondered if he was a hippie. He seemed to ignore me, but I didn't mind as long as I didn't have to talk to him or God forbid, kiss him. He acted like a smart aleck with the other groomsmen (one of which was his brother). I thought long hair on men was a thing of the past. I was disappointed that my cousin set me up with him, but I had to put up with it until the wedding was over. I wondered if he was the type of guy who would do drugs, but I just kept that thought to myself. I was there to support my cousin. At the rehearsal dinner, my cousin presented all the bridesmaids with necklaces as a gift for standing up for her. I was forced to sit next to my long-haired groomsman who was still clowning around with his brother and ignoring me. Although he was underage, he took advantage of the situation and ordered a beer. I just sat and observed.

The wedding day arrived and it was a scramble at my aunt's house with everyone getting ready. I had to remember to take my medication, thyroid pill, and eat breakfast. I was a little uneasy since this was my first time as a bridesmaid. I was hoping I would remember what to do and how to walk. We were ready and the groomsmen arrived at the house minus the groom. The photographer arrived shortly thereafter and took pictures of my cousin alone, then with her mom and dad, then some photos with the bridesmaids. It was very exciting! Everyone was smiling and had happy faces. My cousin and my aunt cried knowing that my cousin was leaving home, but there was little time for that since people were waiting at the church.

The groomsmen arrived with the decorated cars to pick up the bridesmaids. I rode with a couple I didn't really know and my young, long-haired man. I caught the driver looking at me several times in the rear-view mirror, but I didn't know why. I thought maybe my mom told him to keep an eye on me.

We arrived at the church and I met up with my other cousin Mila, the bride's sister. Thank God I had someone familiar I could hang around with. We anxiously waited for the bride to arrive. We all got into place on the church stairs and the wedding ceremony began. I stood next to my groomsman and started walking with my hand on his arm. People were staring at us, and I wondered if they were staring at me or perhaps the look of shock was aimed at my long-haired groomsman. His hair and the tuxedo just didn't seem to go well together. I didn't like walking with him, but I was just hoping to make it through the ceremony without any attention to myself. The wedding lasted more than an hour and then it was on to the reception.

We had a few hours before the celebration started, so we drove to the groom's house to pass some time before going to the banquet hall. I was the youngest one there and they offered me a Coca-Cola, which had plenty of sugar in it. I didn't want to seem out of place, so I sipped on it poured over ice. It was delicious! Nobody paid attention, so I indulged. I had no idea what my blood sugar was, and since I was not feeling bad, I just went with it.

We arrived at the huge reception hall and all the guests were seated at tables. It came time to announce the wedding party and over 250 eyes were on us. It was scary for me. Many people at the reception knew my mom and my deceased, alcoholic father. We were the last couple to be announced before the bride and groom because we were the youngest. I started walking with him and tried not to look at anyone directly. There were too many people and I didn't want to be noticed too much. At long last, we reached the table and I sighed in relief. Next, my cousin and her groom walked to their seats and everyone happily cheered them on. The priest did the prayer and then the couple received the traditional loaf of bread and salt from their parents to represent the body of Christ.

Now it was time for dinner, and at this point I was hungry. I had mashed potatoes, chicken and, of course, ice cream for dessert. I didn't always get to splurge like this. I also had regular 7-Up.

After dinner, the bride and groom began the first dance and the wedding party couples followed. All I had to do was get through that dance and I could be done with my groomsman. As we were dancing, he kept looking away and I thought that was great since I really didn't want to do this either.

My mom's friend Vera was there with her husband and their two girls. They were around my age, so it was great. We were dancing and having fun talking about people at the wedding. They wanted to know all about me and they noticed my long-haired groomsman. We worked the room and then I went back to the head table for a while. I was alone there and my groomsman came over to the table and sat next to me along with another member of the wedding party. As I looked in the other direction, they had poured some alcohol in my drink without me knowing. I continued to drink the 7-Up and then went onto the dance floor to have fun with my new friends, Vera's girls.

I continued to walk around and dance and then as the night wore on, I was giggling up a storm. My mom noticed because I was normally shy and quiet. She asked me if I was okay, and I said "I'm great!" I laughed with the two girls the whole night and towards the end of the evening I had spilled my drink on my dress a few times and thought it was funny. I didn't really care. I was never going to wear that dress again anyway. I never knew if that alcohol in the drink was doing that to me or just the high blood sugar. Later I told my mom what I thought those boys did, and she was in disbelief.

The following day, my cousin had left for her honeymoon and we stayed and visited my mom's friend Vera and her family. I had made it through my first bridesmaid experience. It was not what I expected but in the end, I did have fun. The trip back was another long drive and we made it home safely. I was glad to get home and back to my routine.

After I came home from the trip, I continued to enjoy the summer break and spend time with my friend Beth from junior high. I mostly went over to her house. She lived in a two-story home that was nicely decorated and had a big family that I really admired. One of her brothers was her twin and it just really felt nice to know her.

Looking back at my childhood, I experienced a lot of fear as a result of having diabetes. I felt cheated and deprived of certain foods and had to assume a great deal of responsibility for my health at a very young age. Infections, new diagnoses and surgery were all complicated by the presence of diabetes. My parents tragic split added an additional layer of stress to my life with no father figure in our home, and my mother having to be solely responsible for both of us. I had to forego the carefree childhood that many children experience and learned to be responsible very early in my life. I was fortunate to have such a caring support network with my mother, grandmother and other family members to tend to me. The friendships I formed in grammar school were also invaluable. Those friends helped me forget about diabetes and reminded me that I was cared for despite having a chronic disease – one I worked so hard to conceal.

In adolescence I became more introverted having relocated to a new neighborhood in the suburbs. I continued to hide my diabetes and tried desperately to fit in and be accepted by my new peers. I started to rebel by paying far less attention to my diet, eating more sugar and consequently, I paid the price with high blood sugar. Junior high was difficult as many times I felt harassed feeling like everyone at school knew I had diabetes. Higher blood sugar and puberty impacted my effort and energy to exercise. I experienced more life events that were important and allowed me to build confidence, despite my fears about my diabetes. I started to feel badly about the sugar I was eating and knew it was not good for my health.

Chapter Three

———∽∾∽———

I JUST WANT TO BE NORMAL

BEFORE I KNEW it, the summer was ending and I needed to get ready for high school. I remember Beth being really excited about it, but I wasn't sure what to expect. Was I going to be treated the same as when I was in junior high? My mom and I went shopping for some new clothes which was exciting for me. It felt like I was going away to college. High school was another challenge to face and I had to take my long-time foe, diabetes with me. I wished that I could leave the diabetes behind, but that wasn't an option. It was there 24 hours a day, 7 days a week, 365 days a year.

My first day of high school arrived and I was a wreck. I was on a new bus route and wasn't sure if I would know anyone. Everyone was rowdy and the bus driver let students play their radio including someone who was blasting hard rock. I was just hoping nobody would bother me. I saw some kids that I recognized from junior high, but they were not my friends. Unfortunately, my good friend Beth was not on my bus route. I tried to get a window seat so I could just look out the window. I could not believe how many stops we made, it seemed like we were driving forever just to get to school. The seating was really snug and I could not move around.

The bus arrived at school and most of the kids ran into the building, however I walked slowly to the front door. As I entered all I could think of was how huge this was compared to my junior high school. As I passed the administration office, it was packed with so many students, I felt like I was at a crowded train station. I thought to myself, is this how it's going to be every day? I guess nobody could pick on me if I was hidden in the crowd. Maybe it was a good thing.

I had to hurry and find my new locker and I didn't know where I was going or who to ask for directions. I went back to the administration office to find out. I found it, and then realized I would have new locker neighbors as well. I didn't see them until the next day, because I was focused on how to get to my classes. I felt like a mouse in a maze looking for cheese. The school was three times size of my junior high and was intimidating to say the least. I'm sure my blood sugar was soaring from all the stress.

I heard the first bell for my homeroom class, and I walked frantically through the crowded hallways to get there. I walked in and found a seat, thank God, put my notebook down and just waited for the teacher along with about 30 other students. There were a lot of new faces in the room. The first day was orientation, so I took notes to prevent getting lost. I also made sure I knew where the nurse's office was, just in case. After homeroom I found all my other classrooms and met my new teachers. I made it through the first day and even got on the right bus to go home. It helped that I had recognized some faces from the morning bus, so I knew I was okay. I arrived home and told Baba how it went. She always had something good to eat when I got home. I always looked forward to her special baked goods.

I was exhausted from the day. I wasn't sure yet what I thought of high school, but I knew there would be a lot of running from one class to another every day as well as dealing with the rowdy school bus ride. I had to make sure I ate lunch on time and had plenty to eat so I wouldn't have low blood sugar. This was especially important since I wasn't sure who could help me if I needed it. There was no Mr. Rob there. Even though I should have, I didn't carry any urine test strips with me to school because I didn't want to be found out. I was just hoping I would be treated normally like everyone else. I did wear my diabetic pendant necklace, but I still kept it under my clothes so nobody could see it. I would typically wear another necklace so they would pay attention to the jewelry instead.

The following day I met my locker neighbors. One was a very nice girl named Amy who had a very pleasant personality and I was glad she was my neighbor. I met my other neighbor between classes when we found ourselves at the lockers at the same time. His name was Sam and I remember he was very smiley and cute. I thought about how lucky I was to have a cute guy next to my locker. I would freeze up when I saw him because I was still very shy. I didn't talk much but I smiled a lot and laughed if he told a joke. I did look forward to seeing him.

As the school year went on, I began to get used to everything and made new friends along the way. There were always the cliques in school, and I never really fit in to those. I tried to hang around the nicer girls that I had something in common with. I found a crowd that I would eat lunch with, but they were busy talking with each other. They didn't talk much with me so I sat there and listened to them talk about which boys they had crushes on. I got to know who the boys were, football players, jocks, the burnouts, who was in the choir, and other groups in the school.

Slowly I found my way and where I felt the most comfortable. I never mentioned diabetes, although the girls I sat with started to notice what I would bring for lunch and asked why I never bought anything in the cafeteria. I told them I was on a diet and they asked me why because I was not fat. I always brought a diet soda and always had a can of Hawaiian punch in my lunch bag. I tried to make excuses because I didn't want them talking about me behind my back. Finally, I decided to tell them that I had diabetes. I wondered how I would fare. The girls didn't make too many comments except asking if I had to get a shot every day, and I slowly bowed my head and said, yes. I told them I had diabetes since I was three years old and they said, "Oh you must be used to it by now." That made me angry. How could I be used to painful injections? Every day I after the injection I would rub the site so it wouldn't hurt as much. Then I had to follow a diet to boot. Couldn't they see how badly I wanted to eat the pizza they offered in the cafeteria or how my dream was to have cotton candy?

One of the girl's father was a doctor, so she was more informed. I just wanted to forget I had it and didn't want constant reminders. At home I would eat a piece of candy if I got the chance when no one was looking. How would anyone know if I ate it or not? I would still frequently push the envelope on my diet.

As the months went on, I studied hard to do well in my classes. I was interested in everything, except math - it just didn't sit well with me and I struggled constantly all through high school. I excelled in everything else, particularly art class. I could lose myself in creativity. I liked to draw and paint and learn new types of media. I almost always got an A.

As winter progressed, I still had to wait for the school bus in subzero weather and as a typical teenager, I refused to bundle up. None of the other kids did, so why would I want to look like I was from Siberia? Most of the time I froze, and I wondered later if my thyroid levels were off. My nose was constantly running and my eyes would tear from the cold. I'd barely gotten by that winter, and it seemed longer than usual.

During that season, I broke out in huge red round welts – only on my legs. My uncle Alex came over and was astounded at the size of them. The doctor didn't seem too concerned about it. I can't remember how it was treated, but I pretty much ignored it since it was under clothing anyway. I remember I just wore long socks to cover them. I had to keep the area clean to avoid getting an infection. In a couple of days, the welts went away. It was very perplexing. What had caused them?? I chocked it up as another diabetes "bonus". Why not, it had been responsible for so many other unpleasant things along the way.

My mom bought me an expensive patched suede coat that had real fur inside, on the bottom and along the front. I was the only one in school with a coat like that. We had driven downtown to buy it at a shop my mom was familiar with. She had to put it on layaway because money was still tight. She wanted me to be warm - especially with the hypothyroidism. I remember walking home from school and two older boys from the neighborhood started making snowballs and threw them at my back and hit my beautiful new coat. They were good shots because they hit their target. I couldn't believe what was happening to me. I started walking faster and looking down at the ground until I got to the house, then they disappeared. I greeted Baba, but I didn't tell her boys had been throwing snowballs at me. I wasn't sure if that was their way of making fun of me or harassing me. One was named Neal and the other, Jake. They both lived on the other side of the block. They were quite ornery and unruly. I didn't want to acknowledge them, although I did think Neal was cute. Because I had such low self-esteem, I figured I didn't stand a chance of ever going out with him. Most of the time, I just admired him through the window when he was outside, which was often.

It was Christmas. Baba cooked Christmas Eve dinner and we all gathered to open presents. She set a table and chair with an empty plate for my grandfather as she had for many years. She believed that he would be there to join us for the holiday. I remember receiving a new blow dryer for my hair. I felt great! I had long hair and it took forever to dry it in the wintertime. The blow dryer was a bit on the heavy side – consistent with what was available in the 1970's. My mom took a goofy picture of me holding it next to my head, struggling to hold it. I was so happy. Baba had given me some money and we went shopping for a gift for my mom. I bought her a cowl neck sweater that had three shades of blue. It was so beautiful and I was so happy to give it to her. She really deserved something nice.

We all went to church on Christmas and then we had my cousins over for Christmas Day. My cousins were younger than I and they missed seeing me in the old neighborhood when we lived in a two-flat. They were also trying to get used to their new junior high. My cousin Lina bragged about getting David Cassidy's new album for Christmas. She would come over and we would play it and then record us singing over the music on her Bell & Howell tape player. My uncle Alex worked for Bell & Howell so they would get all the new gadgets.

The holidays were over and back to school I went. At lunch all the girls talked about their gifts and what they did over the holidays, and how they pigged-out. I also snuck some cookies and bakery items we had during Christmas. I wanted to forget I had diabetes. Having those things just made it harder for me to get up in the morning because my blood sugar was soaring until my mom gave me my shot. I don't think she understood why it was so hard for me to get up, but this happened almost every morning. I don't think I ever had a normal fasting blood sugar between 80 and 120. I woke up frequently during the night so hungry I could eat a horse. I dreaded anything to do with restriction. All teenagers rebel, and this was my way. I refused not to eat what I wanted or anything Baba baked. She was truly the baker extraordinaire. When she baked the house smelled delightful, it was a diabetic's dream (or should I say nightmare?). I could smell it long before I got in the house after school. It was always something different all made with yeast of course. I simply couldn't get enough. I was constantly sneaking something when she wasn't looking even though I knew anything with sugar in it was forbidden. When I ate those things I was in heaven, or so I thought. Even though I did this frequently, I could still function. I would go to school with higher blood sugar and even went to gym class and somehow got through it. I was always feeling cold.

As the school year progressed it was always a new day and another dreaded injection every morning. It seemed like my mom kept increasing my insulin. I think Baba told her I was eating sweets and she had noticed that some sections of raspberry cheese coffee cake were missing in the pantry. My mom was trying to help me feel better by balancing my blood sugar, even though I didn't know it or feel it. I did start to pay more attention to my diet. When the blood sugar is normal, the body doesn't crave food as much. I started focusing more on school and just getting through it.

I had another new class; science. I learned about geology and basic scientific concepts. We studied the human body. The teacher brought in cat cadavers that were stripped of their coats with all of the muscles exposed. I remember smelling the preservative they were stored in and it was awful. The next thing we had to do after working with the cat cadavers was to dissect a dead frog, also preserved with the same chemical. That was a one-time deal, we dissected it, kept it for one day and it was gone. Hallelujah! It was really complicated to learn all the parts on something other than the human body, but my teacher wanted us to understand the similarities between human and animal muscles.

High school was definitely harder and more complicated. I was hoping I could keep up, manage the diabetes, and make new friends. Every morning it was even more and more difficult to get up. I was exhausted. I dreaded hurrying in the morning, getting my injection, eating breakfast, then trying to figure out what to wear so I wouldn't be cold, and then try not to miss the bus. Even though these are normal things for teenagers, for me everything seemed to require twice the effort. When I got to class, I was always feeling exhausted until about 10:30 a.m. and then I would begin to wake up. It felt like I was on tranquilizers. If I had gym class in the morning, I just powered through it, trying not to get noticed.

My freshman year was finally over and I made it through. The summer went by fast. In the new school year, I signed up for all the required classes; literature, geometry, gym, and then for electives I chose art, home economics, Spanish, humanities and science. I had a full schedule. I wanted to take Spanish so I could understand some words my mom said in Portuguese. As I found out later, they were two different languages, but my mom was still able to tutor me when needed. On Saturdays I was still going to Ukrainian school to learn about the language, culture, geography, religion and history. I was going to school six days a week then went to church on Sundays so I could hardly ever sleep in. My mom and Baba wanted me to graduate from both Ukrainian school as well as high school. To me it seemed like a waste of time. We always joked around about going to Ukrainian school on Saturday. That should have been my day off!

I turned 15 years old over the summer. Sophomore sounded so much better to me than Frosh. I was still on the shy side so when a cute boy walked by in the hallway I would look down, never making eye contact. I still felt inferior to the other girls because I had a chronic disease. Even though nobody knew about it, I felt like I was wearing it on my sleeve. I remember walking down the hallway towards the cafeteria and there was a very good-looking football player standing there watching all the girls go by and checking everyone out. I was wearing a dress and I felt his eyes roll over me like a bowling ball on the lane. At first I felt embarrassed, then self-conscious, then tiny because of diabetes. I didn't see myself as attractive, so why was he looking at me? He was really good-looking and he knew it. In a way, I was impressed that he was staring at me but I knew I didn't stand a chance with him. After lunch, I had to walk back through that same hallway and he was gone. I remember feeling relieved and disappointed all at the same time. For a split second I was noticed by a hunk. Maybe I wasn't so bad looking after all?

My favorite classes were the ones I found interesting, including art and home economics. Home economics was where we worked on sewing, knitting and crafts. I also enjoyed humanities where I learned about different countries and history. Science was appealing because I was especially curious about human biology.

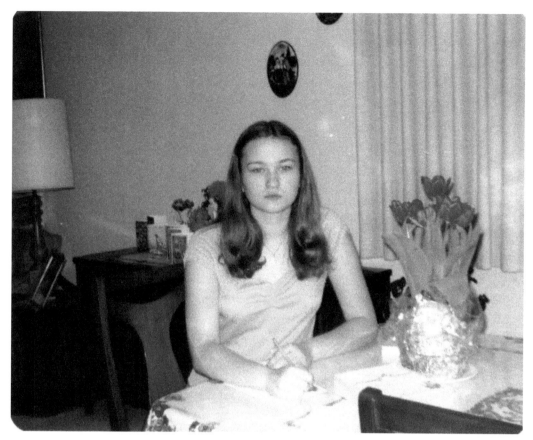

Lucy age 15

It was September and I felt like I was coming down with a cold which I seemed to get frequently in high school. The homecoming dance was just around the corner and some of the girls I knew were going. There was another dance called, "Turnabout" where the girls would ask the boys to go, and I waited for that one. I mustered up the courage to ask a boy named Brock. I wasn't really attracted to him, but he seemed approachable. One day in between classes, I asked him in the hallway and he said "no". It felt like a thousand needles went through my body. That had taken all the courage I had. Trying not to look embarrassed, I said, "okay" and quickly left and looked at the ground while I walked away. I was on the verge of crying, but I didn't because I had to go to my next class. For the rest of the day I was thinking about the rejection and felt, like it was the story of my life. I'm just not normal and so I'm not appealing. I had felt like that all through high school and I never dated anyone. I saw myself as a reject.

Even though I didn't go to the dance, my Sophomore year was busier and more interesting. I enjoyed all my classes, even geometry, though I barely survived it. The next class I had was Spanish. I thought I would do well, and I did. The class was very easy for me since I already knew another language. I felt smart in this class and I think I was the teacher's pet. He called on me frequently to finish a word or sentence as an example. There was a girl named Sara that sat in back of me, and she always said "hi" and talked to me every day. She kept commenting on how easy Spanish was for me and I think she might have been jealous. She was very pleasant and friendly and I liked her as a friend. I would try and help her out whenever she got stuck. I think she got through the class because of me. I went to her house to get together for fun. I was happy to finally expand my circle of friends and get to know someone new. The final exam for Spanish came around, and I felt as smart as I'd ever had in high school. I ended up getting 100% on the exam and finished the class with an A+. It felt great!

In my humanities class, I had two very interesting teachers who actually kept me awake when I was feeling so drowsy from high blood sugar. The class was in the morning, the worst part of my day. By the time the class ended each day, I was intrigued and interested. They taught us about Gothic and Renaissance style buildings through the ages. I enjoyed learning about those things, and still remember it to this day. I became fascinated with Europe and wished I could take a trip to see Italy, France, Spain and more. The teachers incorporated humor into the class and constantly competed with each about which one of them knew the most (in a friendly way, of course). I got an A in that class and learned a lot despite battling high blood sugar misery.

My art class was, by far, the most enjoyable. I truly lost myself in the work and my creativity shined through. I exceled in any type of medium; pencil, charcoal, pastel chalk, watercolor, and screen printing. I also joined art club and I enjoyed every moment. A friend from the group of girls I ate lunch with was also in the class and we became closer. Art made me forget about anything else, it was an escape from reality. I liked being close to God, our creator and, imagined what it was like to create everything we have - the land, skies, water and wind. My talents were a gift from God, there was no other explanation.

I needed to work on a collage for a school assignment. We had a choice of anything we wanted to draw, so I decided I was going to depict Jimmy Carter, our President, and other objects around him. The likeness of President Carter was spot on, and the other images came out very well too.

My collage was nominated to be displayed in the shopping mall with other students as one of the finest in the class for our school district. I was elated! My collage was on display for three weeks. Unfortunately, my family didn't much care for it and it ended up in the basement until it disappeared. I suspect someone, maybe Baba, got rid of it because of the subject matter.

We started indoor gym class since it was getting colder outside. We would play volleyball and badminton indoors during the winter months. I still had to wear that ugly, clingy, knit romper uniform in class that did nothing for my figure, and showed the potholes (atrophic holes) in my thighs from the injections. I just hoped nobody would notice in case my shorts went up. I felt so ugly in that class. I stayed in the back when we were playing so nobody would notice the atrophy in my legs. I tried not to hit the ball if I could help it and let someone else go after it. Needless to say, gym was one of my least favorite classes.

The winter seemed to drag on forever. I froze outside waiting for the school bus, trying to be cool by not wearing a hat or scarf. Consequently, I would get a cold or get some other illness every winter around Christmastime. Fortunately, I had winter break so I didn't have to miss too much school, but I always had to go to my doctor's office and get checked because of my diabetes. Diabetes makes any illness worse, raises the blood sugar and also makes it harder to treat. It always took me longer than usual to recover from colds or any infection. I didn't bounce back easily.

The semester was coming to an end and I received my grades. I got mostly A's, a B, and a C- in math class, but that was normal for me. After winter break the new semester started. I really didn't want to go back. I couldn't wait for spring again because I was always cold. I started crocheting a large blanket at home because I loved creating. It was large enough to fit a king size bed, and at one point I used it to keep me warm while I was still crocheting it. It took me several years to finish it because I would only work on it in the winter months. It was the first of many accomplishments to come. When I wasn't working on homework, or crocheting, I was painting. I had a four-season paint by number kit, which I worked on for several years.

As Spring arrived, we had new activity in gym class, track and field. I wasn't in shape. We had to stretch first to warm up and then run. The teacher punched a timer to see who could run the fastest. Being so out of shape, I couldn't even run slowly! We had to run as a group, so there was added pressure. This class was in the morning, and as usual, I wasn't even awake yet, and had no energy.

As the others started to run, I trailed behind. It was getting harder for me to catch up, and at one point I started to heave. I had a hard time breathing and I felt this cold, burning type pain in my lungs and my legs became rigid, making it hard to move. I couldn't catch a breath, I stayed way behind and ended up walking, gasping for air. My head felt awful, too. I didn't know what was happening to me. When I was a kid I jumped and ran all the time with no effort. Why was I feeling this way? I told the gym teacher I was going to sit out the rest of class, I had to recover. I believe I was running with ketoacidosis in my body which is a combination of high blood sugar and a high level of ketones. I stood by the fence and watched all the other students sprint while I was just holding on to the fence. I felt like a failure. I was embarrassed again. This was one thing my body didn't want to do, or so I thought. While I was not in shape, this incident was likely due to mis-management of my diabetes causing my body to respond poorly to intense exercise. This caused a dangerous scenario.

I dreaded going to track after that. Fortunately, I only had that class for a week or so, then it was on to softball. At least softball didn't require me to move as much or run like a wild horse around a track. All I had to do was try to hit a big ball and run to base. No problem! Nothing could be worse than track. This wouldn't be much exertion at all. Okay, I thought. I can get through this.

I had already participated in several softball games in gym. This day I wanted to get a home run for the team. As I hit the ball the team was yelling for me to slide into base, so I wouldn't get an out. Go! Go! Go! they screamed. Running on pure adrenaline, I remember pushing my leg to stretch into base and as I slid, I felt my right knee go out. It was hard for me to get up. The teacher helped me get to the building and put ice on it. Painfully, I got on the bus to go home. When my mom got home from work, I told her what had happened. She told me to put an ace wrap on it. My doctor told me to just continue with the wrap, there was not much else to do. I had pain on the inside of my knee for a very long time afterward. I was not going to do any more track or softball for the rest of high school.

Final exams came and went for my sophomore year. Another year of school completed and 12 years of surviving diabetes.

Another wedding was on the horizon. My uncle Oleg's brother-in-law was getting married. His fiancé Tammy asked me to stand up in their wedding and I accepted. I was a pro having already stood up in a wedding before. Once again, I wondered who I would be paired with. I was still very shy and though I'd done this before, this would be a challenge for me. I just hoped it would go well. Tammy scheduled all the bridesmaids to pick out dresses on a Saturday after Ukrainian school. Everyone agreed to choose a mint green polyester dress with cap sleeves. I liked this dress - I thought I looked more grown up in it. My mom even bought me shoes to match. Tammy had her wedding shower and received many wonderful gifts. I remember how happy she was that day. The wedding soon followed and I was able to get some sun beforehand. My slightly tanned skin made me look healthier and really looked nice with the mint dress. All the teenage girls were into having a tan using *Ban de Soliel*. Of course, I had to fit in and used it as well.

Everyone seemed to know their part for the wedding rehearsal. It moved quickly and we then went downtown to a famous Italian restaurant for the rehearsal dinner.

Everyone raved about the restaurant. This was my first real meal away from home at a fancy restaurant and I ordered spaghetti and meatballs. Along with a regular Coke, this was a high starch and high sugar meal. I tried not to eat or drink too much. Everyone was older than me, so they were ordering alcoholic drinks. My uncle Paul ordered a Screwdriver and others ordered Hi-balls. When the waiter came to me I remember asking for a screwball. Everyone laughed hysterically. I didn't know what I did wrong. It was the joke of the evening.

The wedding day came. I gave my injection and had a light breakfast. I felt nervous and didn't feel like eating much. My mom was running around pulling things together and asked me if I ate breakfast and I told her I did.

We arrived and all the bridesmaids got their pretty bouquets. They were a little heavy to hold, but I figured it was only for an hour or so. The limo arrived and off we went with our long gowns. I brought my purse with my emergency sugar cubes. I figured I wouldn't need them – I had never fainted since moving to the suburbs. As we arrived at the church we paired up with our groomsmen. Mine was a little older than me, was very cute and looked great in his tuxedo. I was so shy I didn't even know how to start a conversation with him. He was quiet too. My mom wanted to take a picture of us together before we went into the church for the ceremony. The bride and groom were all smiles as they said their vows. I looked across at all the groomsmen. Some of them were sweating as the church did not have any air conditioning. Soon thereafter I began to feel hot but I just thought the room was stuffy. I started looking down at my bouquet. I didn't feel good and felt like my blood pressure was dropping. My mom ran over with a piece of candy and said, "here, here eat this right away." I couldn't open the wrapper. A few seconds later, I fainted and hit the chair behind me. My uncle Oleg ran across the room, picked me up and carried me out the door. Frantically, my mom followed us into the hallway and I started regaining consciousness. I ate the candy my mom had given me and started feeling better. My mom said "The ceremony! You need to go back." I waited a bit before going back into the church and returned in time to exit following the bride and groom. I joined my groomsman and we walked out. Many of the guests came out and asked me if I was okay. It was so humiliating because I didn't want the attention on me. After the ceremony, we spent time at the bride's home before the reception. I made sure to have some food so I wouldn't pass out again. At the reception, I still had people coming up to me asking if I was okay. I didn't want the whole world to know about my diabetes, but they probably did now! I danced a few times and stayed until the bride and groom left. It was a day I will never forget.

It was the summer between sophomore and junior year and I was soon turning 16. I had to take and pass Drivers Education. During the school year, I remember I didn't get much driving experience so I had to take summer school. There wasn't a bus during the summer so I had to ride my bike a good mile to school. It was like climbing a mountain and I would get so out of breath. I was exhausted by the time I got to school. Sometimes hot weather was a factor, but I made it for those two months and finally passed. Mom drove me to get my driver's license. I was excited and I really didn't care if my mom would allow me to drive. To me it was just another accomplishment and soon I was turning sweet 16! I decided to have a birthday party and I invited my closest friends from high school and Ukrainian school. It was a nice party and I got to have birthday cake, but I didn't give myself any extra insulin to compensate. I felt the blood sugar surge after the party, got exhausted and went to bed.

Soon after that my friend Beth got her first job at Ace Hardware as a cashier. I told my mom about it, and she said, "see she's already earning money!" I was a little jealous and I didn't have her to spend time with during the summer. My mom suggested I apply for a job at the mall as Sears Roebuck was hiring cashiers for the summer. I applied, got an interview, and the hiring manager said "are you sure you're 16? You look very young." I said, "I am." She asked me to bring my birth certificate the next day. My mom said "why does she need that?" I told her the hiring manager didn't believe I was 16 years old. My mom just smiled and said "I'll look for the birth certificate." I took it to the hiring manager the next day and she proceeded to hire me. I received a call that they were going to hire me on as a floater and I would work in various departments as needed. That summer I worked in apparel, accessories, paint, live plants, candy, records, and cosmetics, where I ended up spending most of my income. I only worked in cosmetics one time, which is good because I would have spent all my money there. I was only making three dollars an hour but I spent about $40.00 on cosmetics. When I was in the candy department, I had to sell candy to customers. I would have to weigh items and put it in a bag. I don't know how I managed working there surrounded by so much decadence. There was also a machine that made hot, fresh popcorn, and the aroma would fill the entire department. I had a craving every day to eat it, but I had to hold back for the sake of my diabetes and the fact that I was an employee. I remember I had worn high heels working in that department and after a few hours my feet felt like they were on fire. By the end of the day I could barely walk. I also remember getting whistled at when I worked there. I would feel myself turning red but I didn't turn around.

One time, I accidentally spilled candy and I hoped the manager didn't see it and fire me. I was totally embarrassed. I loved having an employee discount and it felt good not paying full price. I took the bus to my job as I didn't have a car yet. I didn't work every day, but it was enough for me and it was always busy. When I worked in the paint department, I noticed it was busier in the summer months, as that was the time of year when everyone tried to get their painting done. I had no clue how to mix paints, but I learned how to do it with the special machine they had. As the customers looked on, I had to know what I was doing. At the end of the summer I was worn out moving from one department to the next and was glad school would start soon. I would miss the money, but I knew that wouldn't last too long. I bought my first pair of real amethyst, 14K gold earrings at a shop I saw the mall. They were fourteen dollars. I had to work nearly 6 hours to buy them. I debated and debated before I gave in and bought them. I immediately put them on my ears and felt so proud and pretty wearing them. It was a good feeling to buy these with the money I had earned. I never lost that feeling for the rest of my life. I never wanted a handout.

It was 1977, and the disco era was in full force. John Travolta starred in Saturday Night Fever and everyone was learning all the dance moves. My Ukrainian school was providing dance classes for a small price and my mom pushed me to join and learn the waltz, fox trot, tango and more. At first, I was reluctant, but then once I got started, I enjoyed the class. I got to dance with a lot of the boys and started considering how they would be as a boyfriend - a silly exercise. I learned the steps more quickly than the boys, and some of them were not good leads on the floor.

It was the end of September and my church was holding a dance that included a live band. My mom had sewn a special dress just for the dance. Since she was a sewing expert, she could make any style that was "in" at the time. As I arrived at the dance, I felt panicky and shy. I hoped I wouldn't feel sick or have low blood sugar, but somehow, I had a lot of energy. The boys from my dance class were there and I kept getting asked to dance all night, often more than once. I didn't realize that I was liked that much, or maybe I was just a better dancer than all the other girls. I think I was on the dance floor for about three hours with a couple breaks. I decided to get a soda in between since I was getting a lot of exercise. Before I knew it, the night was over and some of the boys stayed to tell jokes after the dance for a few minutes. I told them I had fun and would see them in school the next weekend.

My junior year arrived and it was time for homecoming and football season. Some of the girls in my classes were asked to the dance and bragged about the dresses they were going to wear. Nobody had asked me to the dance. After the last fiasco with the turnabout dance, I wasn't that enthused anyway. I figured if someone asked me, that would be fine, but I wasn't going to lose sleep over it. I just continued to do well in my classes. This year my math class was geometry. I actually ended up with a B in the class. Could it be that I was finally understanding math? All my other classes went well and I received mostly A's and B's. I continued to enjoy history and science and all my creative classes, including art. Before I knew it, it was December and the semester was almost over. Right before school break I had come down with a very bad case of the stomach flu. I had a very high fever for several days along with the nausea and vomiting. My blood sugar must have been soaring because I could barely eat anything. Whenever I got up to walk to the bathroom my head was always spinning and as a result spent over a week doing very little. Christmas was spent in bed with the covers and watching TV. I lost quite a bit of weight and felt terribly weak. As I recall, it had been the worst I had ever felt with diabetes. The only thing I could do was to wait out the infection but I had incredible unrelenting body aches that aspirin barely touched. I must have been dehydrated as well. I believe it was God's mercy that spared from a hospital stay. I didn't complain to mom and Baba. They couldn't have known how I really felt. I slowly started to eat and wondered if I would ever get better. I spent the whole school break being sick and languishing around the house.

When school break was over my mom thought I was ready to go back to school but I was still weak. I didn't want to go, but I didn't disobey her. I got on the bus, arrived at school and as I started walking up the steps to go to the second floor, I felt dizzy and out of breath. I still went to class and somehow made it through the day, but it certainly wasn't a day where I learned anything. I was sitting in class with my eyes closed most of the time. The second day I started to feel better and as the week went on, I had improved. After being sick for three weeks, it took another week before I felt 100%. It was a brutal winter with the entire month of January showing below zero temperatures. I suspect that my hypothyroidism caused me to feel even colder. A month later the temperature finally broke and we hit 32 degrees. School went on as usual and after one of the nastiest winters I could remember, spring finally arrived.

I looked forward to Easter and Baba always made it special with her Easter bread and Ukrainian Easter eggs. I had to go to confession before Easter which meant we could not eat or drink anything after midnight. I did not take my insulin injection. The mass lasted about 2 hours and my mom thought I could last without insulin for a while. As we got to church my stomach was growling, but it was a false sense of hunger. I believe my blood sugar was already high and I was burning fat. I remember being dizzy and not feeling well. Mom always carried some juice in her purse for me and she said "have some juice, God will forgive you due to the diabetes." I thought I'd better get something into my stomach to calm it down. Even after the juice, I still felt sick. After confession, we had mass and then had to wait for communion where we all had to eat and drink. I drank the wine and felt it burning down my throat. At this point, I couldn't wait for mass to be over and be forgiven. We got to the car and I gave my injection which burned under my skin, then quickly ate a hardboiled egg with some bread. We went shopping afterwards and I believe the walking likely helped stabilize my blood sugar, though it took all day.

For Easter my family and I went to midnight mass. At 12:00 a.m., the priest announced "Christ has Risen!" and we all walked around the church three times with the Shroud of Christ. After we came home around 3:00 a.m., we had some Easter Bread, butter and a hardboiled egg. It wasn't the right time for me to eat, but as usual I wanted to fit in and be like the rest of the family. It was hard for me to get up in the morning. I suppose I was in ketoacidosis because I was exhausted. That day we had the rest of the family over for Easter dinner. My family always had an abundance of food with deserts galore which tested my willpower. I tried to eat the frosting only on desserts, but with my sweet tooth the temptation was just too great. Inevitably, I had to inject more insulin on the holidays, but I knew my blood sugar was still high.

May arrived and the semester was over, I said goodbye to my junior year. I passed my final exams and qualified to continue on toward graduation. That summer I turned 17 years old. I didn't work during the summer that year as we were going on vacation.

My family decided to visit my aunt on the East Coast for about a week in July. Mom, Baba, and I along with my two uncles drove to the east coast. I remember Baba had packed a cooler with all the food we would need for five people. I also remember eating a bag of potato chips on the road as a snack. Since we were traveling, I used it as an excuse to pig out. My favorite chips were barbecue flavored. I couldn't put them down, and would finish the whole bag before we got to my aunt's house. During the trip, Baba was drinking a lot of water and constantly had to go to the bathroom. We didn't think anything of it since we were on a long trip.

I remember she had been thirsty that whole week at my aunt's house. She continued to eat whatever my aunt would make which included a smorgasbord of food from cabbage rolls, to perogy to borscht and lasagna, to pastries. I never held back when we were on vacation. Every place we visited was full of food. Mom's friend Vera came to visit along with her daughters. We took a day trip to the amusement park where I could have cotton candy, and see the seashore. My cousin drove us there in his Porsche. I got to go on a shopping spree and bought some albums from ELO to Fleetwood Mac. It was a nice vacation that I really enjoyed, and as I reflect back, it was also the most memorable to me.

After a week we drove back home and Baba was still having the symptoms of thirst and frequent urination. My mom was concerned because she knew the symptoms of diabetes and wondered what was going on. I had my own test strips in a glass jar in the bathroom so Baba took one and checked her urine. Her result was

4+, which indicated her sugar level was above 240 mg/dl. Baba had diabetes! She had a very sad look on her face that I will never forget. Baba was in shock and so was my mom. She saw a doctor right away and was diagnosed with Type 2 Diabetes. She could have easily followed a diet to avoid taking medication, but having had a life with food as the central focus, she could not do it. She eventually went on insulin and my mom had to give her injections. Now she had two diabetics to take care of. I believe that Baba saw my example of giving injections and eating anything, so she decided to do the same. Her blood sugar and blood pressure remained high and she was very overweight. I knew now that diabetes ran on my mother's side. I didn't feel as alone despite knowing how this would affect my precious grandmother. I knew the challenges of diabetes and how she would have a hard time following any sort of diet. Baba was 66 and was set in her ways with cooking and eating for so many years. It's wasn't an easy task for her to take the insulin, and watch her food intake. Consequently, her blood sugar was consistently in the 200's.

I had invitations to several parties during the summer, which I gladly accepted. I figured it was a good way to meet some boys, maybe even a boyfriend – I could only hope. A friend of mine from Ukrainian school was having her sweet 16 party and invited me. Nina was tall and slightly overweight and she had a lot of friends in her high school. The party included sweet desserts and fat laden food, potato chips, pretzels, a vegetable tray with dip and hot dogs and hamburgers. It was a teenager's delight. As I arrived at the party Nina greeted me and gave me a hug. I was a little shy since I didn't know any of her friends, but we all sat in lawn chairs and had fun playing games, including charades. I was hoping to find someone I could talk to so I didn't look like an outsider. I managed to talk to several of Nina's friends and I didn't mention to anyone that I was a diabetic. That would be the death of me! After a while Nina had the cake rolled out to the patio and we all sang Happy Birthday to her. Then someone turned on the rock and roll music and we did some dancing. There was a boy at the party that Nina just loved to make fun of. He was originally from Tennessee and had a slight southern accent. He told Nina that he wanted to get to know me. I was taken aback and I wasn't sure if I liked the idea. He wasn't bad looking, and he had a unique persona. He was a bit boisterous and animated, which I found a little intimidating. I was still somewhat shy and timid. As the music played on, he wanted to dance with me. I felt on the spot so I said yes. I figured I would dance with him once and that would be it. I was wrong. He continued to hang around with me and we danced more. As the evening progressed, he took me behind the garage, pushed me against the wall and planted a kiss on me, and more. At this point I didn't even know how to kiss or why I was letting him kiss me in the first place. I did think he was attractive, and now I thought he might want me to be his girlfriend. I didn't even know that much about him however, it was flattering that someone would pay that much attention to me. At the end of the party he asked me for my phone number. I wasn't sure how this was going to work since he lived about 10 miles away and didn't have a car. I gladly gave him my number and hoped he would call.

I told Nina about her friend and that he asked for my number. She said "Him? He's so weird - he's always weird at school. He's from Tennessee." Her words didn't mean much, him kissing me meant more. I didn't hear from him for a few days and then he finally called. I was elated. My first call from a boy, wow, someone actually wanted to talk to me! I didn't know what to say on the phone so I just listened to him talk. At the end of the conversation he said he missed me and I told him the same. We had a phone relationship for a few weeks after that, but we never actually went on a date. He didn't have a car, and he couldn't ask his parents to drive him to see me. When school started, he was a junior and he asked me to go to his homecoming dance. I was floating on air. I was so excited to finally go to a high school dance with someone, even though it was not my school. Nobody knew me there so I didn't have to act any certain way. I immediately told my mom and said, "I need to buy a dress for homecoming!" She knew I was talking to him on the phone for a few weeks already and this would be a double date with one of Nina's friends and his date.

Mom bought me a long mauve-colored dress that was a halter style with bare shoulders and gathers in the front. I felt more grownup, the dress actually made me look older. Of course, my mom was worried about me going to the dance without anyone being aware of my diabetes. I told her I would make sure I had sugar cubes and a can of juice in my purse. I would be sure to eat a good dinner before I was picked up so I wouldn't have to worry.

The day of the dance came and I got myself ready, including my hair and makeup and some nice perfume. My date arrived at the house with the other couple. They met my mom and then we took pictures. He brought me a corsage with pink roses and carnations. I felt like a queen. My date held the car door open for me and we sat in the back seat and held hands. I felt so special, there weren't words to describe it. When we arrived at the dance, we walked in holding hands and I was so nervous, I felt myself turning cold. I wanted to have a nice evening without any problems with my diabetes. I remember as we started to dance a photographer was taking a bunch of pictures. It quickly got very annoying and I wished that he would just go away. I made an angry face at him and wouldn't you know, that image of me was captured. When the evening came to an end, he kissed me good night and said he would call. I said okay, and I wondered if I was his official girlfriend. I asked if I could have a photo of him and he gave me a school picture. On the back he wrote a note thanking me for the memories and that I will always be a good friend. He attended another school and who knew when he could drive out to come and see me. He called me for weeks following the homecoming dance. After a while he said the pictures came back of us dancing at the homecoming dance, and he said I'd looked bored. I was sad that I couldn't have a *real* relationship even though I suspected all along that this would only be short-term. He was my first real boyfriend, and the first one that ever kissed me.

In November, my mom started having problems with her health. A goiter was growing on her neck and her doctor said that it could eventually choke her. Her doctor said the only option was to have it surgically removed. Reluctantly, she agreed to the surgery and was admitted to the hospital within a few days. She was quite worried. What if something went wrong? I remember her surgery took several hours. Once they finished, the doctor said my mom still needed to recover so we wouldn't be able see her that day. When we arrived back the next day, I couldn't wait to see her. Her face was swollen, her neck was wrapped in bandages and she couldn't talk. She was barely recognizable. I reached over to kiss her and she smelled like surgical materials. She knew I was there but couldn't move. Baba started to talk to her. There was a bathroom in her room, and I went in and cried so hard my eyes burned. I was gone for about 10 minutes and mom started asking for me. Baba knocked on the door so I had to pull myself together - I didn't want her to know I was crying. I opened the door and Baba asked, "were you crying?" I said "yes" and continued to cry. My mom motioned with her hands come close, she wanted to hug me. She whispered, "don't cry, don't worry I'll be alright." I was trembling and I wanted to believe it but it was hard after seeing her in such a vulnerable state. I was 17 and I still needed my mom. At the time, I was thinking the worst but eventually she was released from the hospital. The doctor said she would still need some time to recover. She could not move her neck very well for several weeks and had to take thyroid medication and iodine. Now both of us needed thyroid medication to survive.

My boyfriend called me during this time, but I was so distraught I could only think about the most precious people in my life. Since I never got to see him, I didn't give too much attention to that relationship and eventually he stopped calling. I was sad, but I knew it wasn't meant to last.

Several weeks later, my mom returned to her job. She wore a high collar to hide the scar on her neck. She took her medication every day. Baba was finally getting used to giving herself insulin injections, which I taught her to do while my mom was in the hospital. As an observer, I saw all of the changes in our lives as a result of our various health problems. It was very concerning.

I was finally in my senior year of high school. I took some new classes like, interior design, mechanical drawing and typing. There were new things to learn and more ways to be creative while making more friendships along the way. I still had no idea what I wanted to do when I graduated. I was a professional high school student and didn't know what to expect when it was over. Who thought about college? In January, my mom asked me to get some information from the local colleges. I went through all the brochures, but I couldn't see myself doing anything they offered. I was still receiving social security money from my father's death and my mom was insistent that I figure out what my plans were for college. Eventually, we got into a huge disagreement over it. I felt I had just made it through high school with diabetes and she was already pushing me to do more. College was for normal students and I didn't feel normal. I still had a few months to decide before I needed to enroll. I knew I wasn't suited to be an engineer – I was awful in math. I didn't want to be a nurse, I had enough to do just taking care of myself. I had a lot to think about and not that much time.

It was spring of 1979 and I was graduating from high school. Baba was not feeling well. She had been complaining for several days that she had pain under her rib after eating, and soon it became severe. The pain was especially bad when she had a high fat meal. My mom made an appointment for her and the doctor diagnosed her with gallstones that needed to be removed. Surgery was imminent for Baba, and mom was under stress still recovering from her own surgery. We were quite concerned about complications because Baba had other underlying medical conditions, including diabetes, high blood pressure, and obesity. Thankfully, she did just fine. After the procedure, the nurse brought in a jar containing her gallstones and we were flabbergasted on how many there were. Baba was very weak and would need extra care at home.

They put her on a strict diet and after she came home, she lost about 30 pounds. In a few weeks, Baba's scar was healing nicely. It was surprising as diabetics typically do not heal well. She was getting better, but quickly fell back into her old eating habits and baking again.

The final months of high school went quickly. As spring started to blossom, it was time for senior pictures. I elected to have a formal picture as well as some casual outdoor pictures. The photographer mentioned that I posed like a professional model. Naturally, I thought he was just flirting with me. I didn't consider myself a model or beauty at all. I saw myself as a typical 17-year-old girl at best.

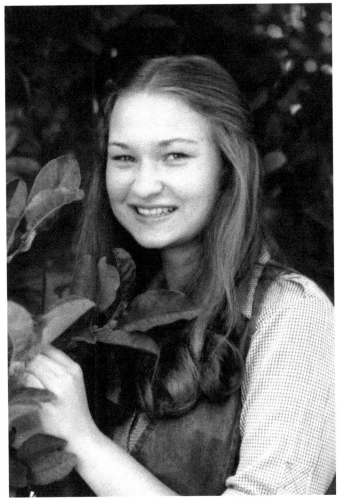

Lucy High School Senior Photo

In a few weeks we received our senior picture proofs. Since I was my mom's only child graduating from high school, it was a big deal, so she ordered quite a few to send to family members. As the school year came to a close, several of us exchanged pictures and wrote in each other's year books. My yearbook was full of personal messages from front to back, several of which complimented me on my sweet, bubbly personality and my amazing smile. I was sad that high school was coming to an end and I would not see a lot of my friends anymore. Most of them were going away to four-year universities and living on campus. I was also graduating from Ukrainian school the same month, so I had two graduations to attend.

Final exams wrapped up and I received the results of my SAT scores. I didn't get a great score and only qualified for community college. I was disappointed but was glad it was over.

Graduation day was ahead. My mom and I went shopping and I bought some Mary-Janes with two-inch heels to go with my graduation outfit. My mom was sure I wouldn't be able to walk in them, but I knew the other girls were getting high heels, and I had to fit in. It was a little overwhelming for me to walk in front of the crowd and I really hoped nothing would happen to me. I remember being nervous and shaking. At graduation, the principal started reading off the names and the valedictorians were first to receive their diplomas and honors. As my name was called, I just looked straight ahead, focused on getting up to the stage with my new high heels. I was handed my diploma, shook the principal's hand and quickly got off the stage being careful not to trip. After all the graduates got their diplomas, we walked back row by row into the adjoining room and met with our families. Mom and Baba gave me a big hug and everyone was excited. After I took off my graduation outfit and hat, I felt sad that high school was over. Once again, I was faced with what to do after high school. A week later I graduated from Ukrainian school. No more classes on Saturday which was a great relief.

In high school, the stakes were higher and the social pressures were tough which made diabetes seem more difficult. I had low self-esteem and was having to face judgmental new peers, and an even harder time thinking about interacting with or dating boys. High school had a more complicated schedule, and I tried to focus on getting good grades so I could graduate. Revealing my diabetes to my peers was especially hard. Managing my blood sugar was a constant struggle and having low energy really impacted my health.

Dating was the scariest time for me. I wondered if or when I could reveal the chronic condition I'd been managing. Then once revealed, whether the other person would have the maturity to accept and support me or would instead see it as an inconvenience.

As my mom and grandmother started to have medical issues it was very unsettling. I was the only one that was supposed to be ill! Life was about to get more challenging as new diagnoses and events continued to unfold.

Chapter Four

COLLEGE BOUND

MY MOM WANTED me to go to the nearest community college, which meant I would need a car. We went to get some brochures and I wasn't really interested in much. My mom pushed me, but it was very hard. With her having to pay for my schooling I felt I needed to make a good decision and one where I knew I couldn't fail.

One day that summer, my mom said it was time for me to get a car. I didn't really ask for one, but I thought it would be great to get a nice Buick Regal like I had in drivers ed. Of course, that was a luxury car at the time, but I still dreamed about it. I was a little afraid to drive, but because I had not had low blood sugar for a very long time, I didn't allow it to bother me. In a way, the independence of having my own car made me feel like I wasn't diabetic anymore and I could be just like everyone else my age.

My mom and my uncle and I went looking for a car. He told the salesman I was looking for a car at a good price. The salesman mentioned he had a nice 1979 Ford Fairmont Futura. It was a demo with low mileage and I could get it at a great discount. I liked the car and it drove nicely with its luxurious red velvet seats and gray exterior. After we got the car, I drove it home. As soon as I parked it in the driveway, I immediately sent my mom inside for the camera so she could take a picture of me behind the wheel.

Now that I had wheels, my mom told me to get a summer job until college started. I went to the local mall and applied at an apparel store for plus-sized women. I already had experience working at the mall so it was familiar to me. I liked having my own money again. I made sure to save some of it so I could purchase my school books. My job responsibilities included cleaning up the dressing rooms, keeping the store organized and checking out customers at the service desk. Frequently, I would feel tired at work so I would sit down when nobody was looking. I suspect it was because my sugars had been high.

I had to see a school counselor to try and figure out what courses I wanted to take in college. The counselor told me a lot of students out of high school didn't yet know what they wanted to do. After looking through the college brochures, the only thing I found interesting was fashion design/fashion merchandising. My mom wasn't a fan of my selection but gave in and enrolled me in community college for the next two years.

It was the end of August, 1979 and classes were starting. The first day of college, I drove my car and parked in the huge outdoor parking lot. It was a long walk to get to the building. The first day was orientation and I needed to get acquainted with the campus and all the various buildings. I lived in the upper Midwest and the distance from the parking lot and between buildings was going to be pretty tough in the wintertime. There was nothing I could do, I had to go.

The first day of class I met the students and the teacher and we all had to say something about ourselves. I had nothing much to say, just that I enjoyed fashion. I felt alone, I didn't know anybody, and I didn't know if they were nice or not. I never mentioned I had diabetes. A few of the women in class were in their forties and decided to go back to college after having raised their kids. It was different going to school with students that were my mom's age.

One of the segments of the course was about learning to draw designs on figures. The instructor told us to get a book from the library on human anatomy, so we could study the muscles and figure out how to draw the human body on paper. Then we could develop our own creative designs and see how they would look and flow on the body, just like a designer. As I started to look at the muscles in the anatomy book, I found myself interested in the science behind it. It was really fascinating, and I hadn't learned human anatomy in high school during biology class. I did finally learn how to draw figures by studying the book. One day, the instructor brought in some slinky qiana fabric which was something new on the market. There was a contest and the student who came up with the best design for the qiana would win the fabric. This was a challenge and above all else, I'd hoped to "out design" those two students in their forties. My design was a dress with raglan flouncy sleeves. For the focal point, it had two panels that tied in the front forming a knot. I showed my mom who was an experienced seamstress, and she really liked it.

The instructor took home all the designs, graded them, and brought them back for class. I was anxious for the results. She went over some of the good designs and showed us the highlights. Then she named the runner up, who was one of the older women.

When she said "this is the winner!", low and behold it was my design. She loved the way it hung and flowed and felt it was perfect for that qiana fabric. I was so happy because though I wanted to, I never expected to win. This was more of my creative talent that I had always enjoyed expressing. The teacher asked me if I was going to make the dress and I told her I wasn't sure, but I was thrilled about having the winning design.

As the semester went on, I did well in class, and made friends with another girl who was going into fashion merchandising. She wanted to manage a store after graduation. I already had experience of working in retail, and knew it wasn't going to be a career for me. I also realized that in order to make it big in the fashion industry you need to have all the right contacts.

I started to think a lot about the anatomy book I borrowed from the library. After learning about the complexities of the human body and having diabetes for almost 16 years, I wanted to learn more. I wanted to know what made the human body work, and maybe I could find out how to feel better in the process. When the semester came to a close, I told my mom I didn't think I would really succeed as a designer and I wanted to be a scientist or at least give it a try. In order to pursue that, I had to transfer to another community college because this one didn't have the courses I needed. I think my mom was happy that I came to my senses and wanted to study something that would prepare me to get a good job after graduation.

After the semester ended, I was going to transfer to another school that offered a two-year degree as a Medical Lab technician. I would have to take some heavy-duty science classes as well as chemistry. I wasn't sure what I was getting into.

As summer approached, I got a job working at the same company as my mom in their parts department. I got the job easily since she already worked there as a keypunch operator. The company made charcoal grills and I handled filing and paperwork. The office where I worked had a window view of the guys in the parts department working with boxes and sorting parts for shipment. It was an enjoyable job and we all had fun most of the time. Nobody really took their job too seriously because we were all college students making extra money. Sometimes the guys would make faces at us through the window and we would make faces back at them. They played jokes on us and even locked me in the bathroom one time by tying a rope on the doorknob to a nearby pole so I couldn't get out. I admit I didn't think it wasn't funny, they knew I had diabetes. This was the first job where people knew I had diabetes. I didn't want to be left in there without my purse and emergency food. I remember yelling at them to open the door and pulled furiously on the doorknob. Subsequently, one of the girls in the office saw what was happening and they let me out. Boys will be boys! I was a nervous wreck after coming out of there and they were all reprimanded for it.

They hired a new guy in the parts department where I worked. He did a lot of lifting, putting heavy boxes on shelves and always seemed to sweat buckets. His name was Tim and he was working there during college summer break. I used to see him having huge milk shakes for lunch and several whoppers for lunch and thought, I wish I could have a large milk shake like that for lunch. I never even touched a milk shake but I was really jealous to see someone else have one. One day he ended up in the hospital. I asked what happened and they told me he was hospitalized for ketoacidosis. What? I couldn't believe it. Tim was a diabetic? He was clearly ignoring his diet. His blood sugar was 800 mg/dl and I had told the girls in the office how he could have died. I might have been the only one that really understood what that meant. I was in shock and I hoped he would make it out alive. I was really concerned and constantly asked how he was doing. Thankfully, after a few days they were able to stabilize his blood sugar and he returned to work. I was happy and relieved to see him back at work and told him I was a diabetic too. I asked him why he ate so much and had a large milk shake with a meal. He said "its fine, I work hard so I have to eat." Even though I'd told him how serious this was, he didn't really appear to care. Soon Tim ended up in the hospital again for the same thing. This time they discovered his kidneys were compromised so he had an even longer stay. I continued to watch him abuse his diet and constantly sweat buckets. I just shook my head. He was in denial.

One of the big bosses at work was having a pool party and everyone was invited. When I arrived, I remember being stunned by the size of his home and his 60-inch TV set. This man wore several big, gold chains and he was exceptionally nice. The pool was magnificent. I noticed Tim and his girlfriend frolicking in the pool and watched as he lifted her on his shoulders. I walked over and told him to be careful, and also told his girlfriend to watch him. I found a spot and sat on the edge of the pool in the sun, I didn't want to be getting in and out of the water because it made me feel cold. I'm sure my hypothyroidism had something to do with it. As I sat in the sun, one of the owner's sons approached me and started to talk to me. He was around my age, and we started talking about Tim and how he ended up in the hospital twice. In that moment I was feeling comfortable and told him I was also diabetic. He asked me if I was having a good time, I said "yes, of course." I started talking about how diabetes is hard work and that Tim needed to be taking care of himself. It took a lot of courage, but I told him how long I had diabetes. He said "I'm so sorry you have diabetes, I wish you didn't." It felt really good that he cared and had empathy for me. I almost wanted to say, "Will you marry me?", but it was just a passing thought.

After the party, I came home and told my mom about the party. I told her I liked the owner's son because he felt badly that I had diabetes. Someone besides me thought it was awful to have diabetes. It was a joy to know that and it really put a smile on my face. I thought about it for days after because it made such an impression on me. I was hoping I would marry someone like him, but I knew he was untouchable. My mom had a very good job there. She worked with computers and not in the factory. We had good insurance which was very important to us.

I kept in touch with my friends from high school and Ukrainian school after graduation. I always wanted to have friends and not be isolated. I kept in touch with my friend Abby from my typing class, we wrote letters while she was away at college. I also called Nina frequently and asked about my homecoming date and how he was doing.

As my summer job ended, I started attending a new community college in a Medical Lab Technician program. It was a different school again, and I felt more alone than ever. I thought college was so callous and impersonal and everyone seemed to keep to themselves. I purchased all my books which included Human Anatomy and Physiology, Microbiology, Organic Chemistry and English. I had about 17 hours of courses; it was a heavy load. I was going for an Associate's degree which would take two years. I was hoping I would do well and that diabetes would not get in my way.

During the first few days of classes, I tried to get to know some of my classmates. I enjoyed the courses but I had some serious reservations about the Chemistry class. It involved math and that had never been my best subject. All my classes were during the day, so I had lots of studying every evening.

One day in Biology class the instructor started talking about diabetes and what could happen with the pancreas. There was a girl named Jean who I had told about my diabetes just prior to the class. As the instructor started to explain what happens in someone with diabetes, the thirst, the weight loss, the destruction of the islet cells in the pancreas, I felt like she was talking about me. My soul was screaming from the inside as if I was being criticized. She kept repeating how important it was to keep the blood sugar levels as normal as possible and discussed diabetic complications. I was a jittery wreck just sitting and sliding in my chair listening and I wanted to cry. Then the instructor asked the students to share what they had learned. One student asked if she could get diabetes since her sister had it. The instructor advised there was a 50/50 chance. The girl said quietly under her breath "I hope I don't." At that point, I was ready to just get up and walk out. I kept looking at the clock to see how many more minutes were left until the class ended. My heart started to beat faster and I felt like I was on trial in a courtroom. It upset me that the instructor was going on and on about diabetes. Jean just sat next to me and didn't say anything. After class she invited me to come over to her house for a visit and I accepted her offer. She lived in a very nice neighborhood. We didn't really talk about my diabetes and when I came over, she offered me bread rolls and cheese. I took a few bites and then left the rest on the plate. I wanted to eat all of it, but the diabetic discussion from that class was pounding in my head. We had a good time and I met her family and her fiancé. I was a bit jealous on the inside, but I showed happiness for her on the outside.

Microbiology class required us to memorize a great deal. The instructor I had was quirky. She had a southern drawl and she seemed to pay more attention to me than the other students. She noticed I was wearing a medical alert bracelet, and I had to tell her I had diabetes. We learned how to use the electron microscope the first week, how to focus, and the appropriate magnifications to use on everything from cells to bacteria. As I looked at the microscope and asked her for directions, she took my hair and swept it behind my shoulders. It was almost like she tried to comfort me and I sensed she felt bad I was diabetic. It made me uncomfortable that she did that because I didn't like anyone touching me. I didn't say anything and brushed it off. The microscope was an interesting tool to me and I hoped I could change people's lives by learning about microorganisms. One of the first tests we had in class was to get our own urine sample and look at it on a slide under the microscope. The instructor told us to look for certain things, how many cells were normal, the color, the specific gravity, and to look for calcium oxalates or casts. Casts could be found in the urine of people who had kidney damage and I was praying I would not see any casts. God answered my prayer. My urine was normal. The instructor said that she did have a student in her class who discovered casts and it was determined that she was in kidney failure. It was very difficult for me to hear about those things. I asked if the student was alright and she said the class saved her life. I reluctantly asked the instructor if this could happen with diabetes. She said yes.

For the next assignment, we had to bring in a urine sample from one of our family members. I chose Baba, since she also had diabetes. Baba found this to be a pain because it required a 24-hour collection period. When I looked at the jar, I immediately saw that there was a chalky white substance that had settled to the bottom. Baba thought it was unusual and she asked me what it was but I didn't know. I asked the instructor what the substance was and she said it was calcium oxalates. This is pulled from the bones and excreted in the urine. She said that this was typical in people who ate a lot of meat – an indication of diet. I wasn't sure what to think, was Baba in danger?

In microbiology, I really enjoyed learning about the cells and what was normal. The next assignment was an examination of our own red blood cells. All the students had to prick their fingers and put blood on a slide. When I first saw the red blood cells, they looked like little donuts but without the holes. The instructor said that oxygen flows in and out of the cells, through a thin membrane in the middle, and that is also how we receive nutrients from food. My cells were tiny but there were a lot of them there. I asked why they were so tiny and she asked, "do you have anemia?" and explained that anemia was a result of low iron and could cause fatigue. This made a lot of sense to me because I constantly felt tired which I attributed to high blood sugar. I was a little concerned, but she said "it's likely individual to you and you should not worry about it." I immediately went to the pharmacy after class and bought Theragran-M, a multivitamin with iron and I started taking one every day. They were expensive, but I didn't care. I just wanted to feel better. We had to memorize what the different cell types were and what their function was for our first exam. I received an A and was anxious to learn more.

The next semester was more intense. This was where I had to learn about all the different types of bacteria, and how to recognize them both in a petri dish as well as under the microscope. I had my mom help me memorize the different names from staphylococcus to streptococcus to spirochetes to pseudomonas aeruginosa. I also had to know what types of diseases they caused. When I learned about the ones that were sexually transmitted, I was horrified that one person could pass it to another. I vowed to save myself for marriage as I had enough problems to deal with diabetes.

During the late fall, my friend Abby came home from college. I invited Abby to meet up with some friends as bunch of us were going on a hayride. I was interested in getting to know a guy I had met at a previous get together. They had some wine on the ride and everyone was taking sips. As the bottle came to me, I took a couple of sips, but not because I wanted any, I just wanted to fit in. Abby saw a guy on the hayride that went to the same college as she did and he seemed to like her. It was a fun time and we all joked around. The guy I liked asked me for my phone number.

A few days following the hayride I started to feel sick. I had a fever and chills and I had to miss school. It turned out to be a severe case of bronchitis and I had to take a heavy dose of penicillin which was not easy to swallow. I had high blood sugar, I couldn't eat much and lost weight. At one point I felt a squeezing sensation in my diaphragm (the area just above my stomach) and experienced terrible muscle twitches all over my body. It felt like someone was pulling hard on my muscles. It took a month but I did finally recover from the bronchitis. Unfortunately, the muscle twitches continued and I had to go back to class with this bothersome problem.

I successfully finished all of my classes for the semester. I started to read books about muscle twitching and anemia in the hopes of finding out how to address it. I checked out various books at the library and read up on symptoms. I found out that muscle twitches were caused by a lack of magnesium so I bought some at the local health food store and started taking it. I didn't get any relief, but it's possible I may not have been taking enough. I learned later that high blood sugar drains the body of minerals including sodium and magnesium when the body is in ketoacidosis. I was on the right path, so I continued to take the supplements if I could afford them. I remember taking the Theragran-M throughout my early 20's.

It was 1980 and for the first time in my diabetic experience a new device, Accu-Check, was approved to check precise levels of blood sugar. The meter and the required test strips were expensive, however this device allowed me to quickly assess my blood sugar level which often fluctuated a great deal because I was a brittle diabetic. I introduced Baba to the meter and strips as well, but she didn't use them consistently. As I approached my twenties I needed to find a new physician, – an endocrinologist that treated adult diabetes and hypothyroidism.

I was gaining more knowledge about supplements including vitamin B complex. I decided to try it and bought some from the health food store. I took them for a couple of days with no problem. On the third day, a flush came over me and I broke out in hives. I felt like I was going to faint. My mom rushed me to the emergency room and it appeared that I had an allergic reaction to something in the vitamin B complex. I was given epinephrine which made my heart feel like it was coming out of my chest. The ER doctor then gave me Benadryl which made me tired. The hives went away, but I felt awful from the drugs for the rest of the day. Needless to say, I stopped taking the vitamin B complex.

Occasionally, I would notice that my heart seemed to skip a beat. I made an appointment with a cardiologist and he ordered some tests. He said it sounded like I had a heart murmur. I had an EKG done and an echocardiogram. After a few days the results came back and I was diagnosed with mitral valve prolapse. The doctor said it was it was a mild case, it wasn't serious, and they would keep an eye on it. He said many young women that are tall and thin tend to have this problem. I was the thinnest ever. One more health problem I had to add to my list. With this condition it was important that I learn to control anxiety so my heart would not beat fast and skip. I was also aware that a person can faint from mitral valve prolapse which really concerned me.

The second semester started and I had to take inorganic chemistry, which turned out to be a night class. The instructor in this class was ineffective. He did not explain a lot in class. His teaching style was for us to read the chapters and come to class, with almost no instruction. I didn't care for his approach and I had difficulty learning or understanding much of anything.

As the semester continued, I excelled in the other Medical Lab Technician courses. In human anatomy we were shown a cadaver preserved in formaldehyde and the smell was almost unbearable. We studied the skin and muscles that were exposed in certain parts of the body. The face was covered, and we were not allowed to look at it. Most of the students stood silent and let the instructor talk. I was trying to hold my breath as much as possible for the 10 minutes we spent before leaving the room. It was a bizarre experience.

I did very well in all the courses except chemistry. After the final exams were graded, it turned out that I failed inorganic chemistry. I was upset, and felt it was due to the incompetent instructor. I had passed all the other difficult lab courses. I was told by the college that in order for me to continue in the program, I needed to take the first year over. This was extremely upsetting because I had only failed one course. I couldn't imagine taking all those courses over again. I told my mom and she said, "you need to finish college." I met with the school counselor and he told me that I could transfer my credits to another school. I told him I would look at the previous school I attended and see what was possible. As it turns out I could easily transfer my credits to a Registered Nurse program. However, I would still need to go another two years and I simply couldn't afford it. The counselor then told me about a new program called Medical Office Assisting. I could transfer my credits and finish it up in one year. That sounded good, but I had really hoped to do scientific work. At this point, I felt I had no choice but to finish with the Medical Assisting. I agreed to sign up with the program and hoped I could graduate within one year.

During the summer of 1980 we wanted a nice vacation and my mom decided to go to Florida. This was my second time on an airline and I had to remember my medications; insulin, syringes and thyroid medication along with my supplements. I was able to carry everything on the plane with no restrictions, I just needed a doctor's note that I was a diabetic and needed everything with me.

When we arrived in Orlando, Florida, I was amazed. It was hot and beautiful with tropical plants that I never saw before. We checked into the hotel and had a view of the city. I didn't mind, I just wanted to explore Florida since I had never been there. We had to eat out at restaurants and the first meal we had was lunch at IHOP. I didn't know what to order so I chose the spaghetti with marinara sauce along with a salad. I ate about half and then my blood sugar went soaring, which explained why I started to feel sick to my stomach. I couldn't eat anymore, so I just finished the rest of my Tab soda. We went shopping afterwards and walked around town which was the best thing I could do.

I told my mom that I wasn't feeling well. I had some pain in my vaginal area and I felt nauseated. When I went to the bathroom, I noticed fresh blood. It wasn't normal. She checked with the hotel to see if they had a physician, and they said no, but they could refer me. My mom called the doctor's office and asked if I could get in immediately as we were from out of town. The nurse scheduled an appointment that afternoon and I was seen. I felt really ill, like nothing I had experienced before. I told the doctor I had bleeding from the vaginal area and he asked when I'd had my last period. I wasn't due for another few weeks so I had to have a vaginal exam. Even though I was 19, I had never had one before. As the doctor examined me, I started to scream and cry from the pain. My vaginal walls were red, inflamed and bleeding. The doctor said "dear, you have a nasty yeast infection." I asked for more information and he said "diabetics get this frequently and antibiotics exacerbate the problem. The yeast feeds on sugar, antibiotics, and hormones and it gets worse and worse." I knew I had the itching and burning for a long time, but my symptoms had come to a head and I was really paying for it. I hoped this wouldn't ruin my vacation. The doctor wrote a prescription that I had to use daily. The medication burned like crazy and I went to bed crying in the hotel room. I imagine I must have had this for years without ever treating it, and it finally became a disaster. I was more upset than ever at having diabetes. I wondered if I was the only one who had ever experienced a yeast infection this severe. As the week progressed, I started to feel much better. Thank goodness the doctor diagnosed this, but too bad it took a trip out of state to finally get resolved.

We decided to go to Daytona Beach. I knew a lot of college kids went there for spring break. The weather was really hot and I wanted to dip my feet in the ocean, but I didn't go swimming. My mom loved to sunbathe. I had fair skin and light eyes but I still wanted to get some sun and look like I had been on vacation. I laid on the beach during peak hours and I thought I would just get darker. I felt the sun penetrating my eyes, even though they were closed. I had some tanning oil on me, but without any SPF which really wasn't available then. We got back to the hotel and had a light dinner. After dinner I started to feel sick, got the chills and I realized I had a severe sunburn. I laid in bed with a fever and I couldn't stop shaking. I had to see a doctor, but there wasn't one available at the hotel. My mom took me to the local emergency room. What a vacation! I was diagnosed with sun poisoning and second-degree burns. They put some cold cloths on me to cool down the burns, but it didn't help much. They also used Silvadene cream. That seemed to help for the moment and I would need to use it for the rest of the vacation. Slowly the chills subsided and I was told to stay out of the sun, which was difficult in Florida. My skin started to peel everywhere and it was awful. Toward the end of the vacation my mom bought me a pearl ring at Disneyworld. It was the happiest moment I had on that trip.

After we arrived home from Florida, my aunt called and said my cousin Mila who was about 8 years older than I, was getting married. The wedding was going to be in

New Jersey and my aunt asked my mom if I could stand up in Mila's wedding as a bridesmaid. I agreed because after all, this was family. Mila ordered the bridesmaid dress for me and then sent it via mail. The dress was a peach color with flowers and pleated from the waist down. I really didn't care for the polyester dress. It also had straps that tied at the shoulders to hold it up. The wedding was going to be in August, so I had a few months to tailor it, if needed.

Mom went back to work and I got a job working part-time in a women's clothing store as a cashier. The summer went by quickly and during my spare time I would meet up with local friends. I slept over at a friend's house one weekend and we went shopping the following day. I had my medications, Accu-Check meter and sleepover bag with me. This was the first time my friend saw me giving myself an injection and pricking my finger to check my blood sugars. My friend wasn't the greatest cook. She made some burnt toast and then she threw a whole egg into boiling water and it burst. I asked her for some orange juice which luckily she had in the house. I knew I had to have something to eat otherwise I could faint with too much insulin and not enough food. After breakfast, we went shopping and I checked my blood sugar. It was elevated likely from too much orange juice. I had to give myself another injection. We were in the car and I drew up the insulin from the vial into the syringe. My friend said, "don't show that, someone might think you're a drug addict." I said "I don't care, I need to have this," and I continued, pushing down my jeans enough to inject the insulin into my stomach. My friend looked at me awestruck. She said "I could never do that." I said, "you would if you wanted to live. This is what I do every day." She said "well, you must be used to the shots by now." This aggravated me. Does anyone get used to pain? I said "no, I will never get used to the shots." After the injection we went to the mall and I bought some fast food for lunch. I tried to stick with a hamburger as I knew approximately how that would fit into my diet, along with a diet soft drink. I was just happy that I had a friend who accepted my condition and thought of me as a friend first and a diabetic second. However, I don't think she really understood my dilemma with this disease. I think she just admired me for being so skinny.

Mila's wedding was coming up and I had my bridesmaid dress tailored to fit. Baba, mom, my uncles and I drove out to New Jersey. As we drove on the Turnpike I remember someone had spray painted on a bridge "Who Shot JR?". The television program, Dallas that I watched every week with Baba, starred Larry Hagman who played JR. His character had been shot since he was hated by so many people. After a 16-hour trip, we finally arrived. My aunt greeted us and everyone helped with the suitcases. Mila had many out of town guests. Her fiancé was from Pennsylvania and we met him for the first time. He seemed nice and was a good match for my cousin Mila.

We all settled in and enjoyed a large dinner that my aunt probably spent all day making. I never went hungry at her house. Baba and my aunt loved to be in the kitchen conversing. By now, I knew what to expect after standing up in a few weddings. I was going to be standing up with my cousin Sam, Mila's brother. I was hoping for someone else, but at least I wouldn't be nervous.

The following day was the wedding. Mila looked so calm like she didn't have a nervous bone in her body. I, too, felt calmer at this wedding. I knew that I would be standing up with a family member who knew I had diabetes. I still had no appetite before the wedding, but I had some breakfast, including orange juice. Nobody had time to make a big breakfast but my mom wanted to make sure I ate. I told her I had.

The limo arrived and we were off to the church. All the girls were smiles, including myself. The wedding was in late August, so it was still summer and the small church got warm. About 45 minutes into the ceremony, I started to feel sick like I could potentially faint. I let my mom know and she and my uncle walked me out the back door. My mom was furious and asked me again if I had eaten anything that morning. There was a bench close by so I sat down with my mom while my uncle got some soda for me from the church hall. It seemed like it took him only a minute to get back. Since I was feeling better so quickly they told me "you need to go back in and finish the wedding". I sensed that my mom was irritated that this had happened to me again at a wedding. She kept asking if I was okay, and I really did feel much better. I entered through the back door and quietly made my way to the front with the rest of the bridesmaids. They all looked at me and I told them I was okay. At least this time I didn't fall down. As expected, I had people coming up to me after the ceremony to ask if I was alright. Once again, I felt diabetes was making me stick out like a sore thumb, and I was embarrassed. I wasn't doing this to get attention.

All of us drove back to my aunt's house after the wedding to take more pictures and have some snacks. I was assured there would be a lot of food at the reception. I had no doubt because this was a Ukrainian wedding. In terms of food, it was comparable to an Italian wedding – food was everything. The only thing I looked forward to were the desserts and the wedding cake. This was forbidden for me, so of course I wanted them. This was a great chance not to think about diabetes and indulge. It was my cousin's wedding, so why not?

The reception was huge and it was fun. I thought I would enjoy myself eating, but instead I had fun seeing my cousins, laughing, dancing and not even thinking about indulging too much. I had enjoyed spending time with my family since I didn't get to see them very often. I danced the first dance with my cousin and then took off on my own mingling with more people my age and talking about my drama show at church. I had some Seven-Up and walked around with the drink like it was a cocktail. I remember my cousin asking me if it was an alcoholic drink, and I said yes. A sugary soda was just as poisonous to me as alcohol, but it felt good to pretend I was normal and walk around with a drink. I felt cool. The reception went on until about 2:00 a.m., and I had to get up in a few hours for my insulin injection. Diabetes never left. I could always count on it to be there the next day and I that I had to take care of it. In a few days we had to make the long trip back home.

The following weekend, my friend Abby invited me to her friend's party. I was excited to go. I was tanned from summer and I thought I looked good. After my cousin's wedding, I was in the party mood.

I arrived with Abby at the party and everyone there was holding an alcoholic drink, and some were smoking. I was introduced to some new people and I started talking to one guy who was short and skinny, I remember he had a friend standing next to him who I found to be really attractive. The guy I met on the hayride was also there and came over to talk to me. After the party got started I danced with him, but my focus was on that other guy I thought was so good looking. His name was Jesse. I started asking around to find out more about him. The girl who was having the party said she knew him and I told her how I thought he was so attractive. She told his friend, the short and skinny guy. After about 10 minutes, Jesse approached me and started talking to me. I felt my flight or fight reaction kick into gear. My hands were sweaty, my heart was fluttering, and I was panic-stricken. I was hoping I could remain calm and secure in myself. Jesse did most of the talking, telling me all about how smart his friend was. I asked Jesse where he lived and what he did for work and he told me he was a mechanic. He seemed quiet and there wasn't much conversation thereafter. I stood next to him for the rest of the night, sipping a coke. It was after midnight when Jesse asked me for my number. I didn't have a pen, and the hostess could only find a yellow marker and a white piece of paper. I was hoping he would be able to read it and would call me. After the party I was ecstatic. I told Abby what happened and I kept envisioning my first date with him. I was already infatuated, and even though I had just met him, I thought about marriage and kids. It was a little premature, but what did I know.

After three days, Jesse called me. I remember answering the phone on one and a half rings. I was jumping out of my skin with joy. I was hoping I wouldn't say the wrong thing. We talked for a while and then he asked me if I would like to go to dinner. I said yes, of course, and after we hung up I ran and told my mom all about Jesse and his call. I told her that I thought he might like smoking marijuana, but I wasn't sure. She immediately said she didn't feel it was safe for me to go on a date with him. I kept trying to convince her I would be all right, and that he was a friend of a friend of Abby's. Even though my mom really didn't approve, she let me go on the date because she didn't want me to be isolated. For the rest of the week all I thought about was my first date with Jesse. I could barely contain myself. I ate very little, but the high adrenaline made my blood sugars soar over 200 mg/dl every day.

Saturday night came. I wore my best dress, wonderful perfume, and my makeup and hair were perfect. Jesse picked me up and he was wearing an attractive shirt and slacks. The restaurant he chose was the nicest place I had ever been. The design was unusual with a tilted glass ceiling and it was romantic. I ordered a well-done steak, mashed potatoes and a salad. Jesse ordered the same, along with some red wine. I told him I didn't drink, so I ordered a coke instead. As we waited for the dinner, all Jesse kept saying was how beautiful I was. Flattered, I smiled and thanked him many times. He would not stop staring at me. All I could do is stare back at him. I felt so lucky to be on a date with such an attractive guy, but at the same time I didn't know how I should act. I was nervous, but played it cool and didn't show too much emotion. I was actually more scared than anything. I just hoped I wouldn't faint or feel sick because Jesse didn't know I was diabetic.

When dinner arrived, I ate only half of my meal. Jesse asked if there was something wrong. I said it was just too much food for me, but that it was delicious. The whole time I kept reminding myself that I can't over eat, and I can't under eat. I want to feel good during our date. I thanked him for the meal and then we drove to a local park with a lake and just sat in the car and talked. He complimented me on my eyes, and told me how beautiful they were. I kept thinking how jittery I was. He leaned in to kiss me and he was just the best kisser I thought. I couldn't stop kissing him. My heart was beating out of my chest. After a while I felt more comfortable, and my heart went back to normal. We went back to kissing some more and holding each other. I was so infatuated and I felt enveloped by him. I asked him if he did drugs and he told me he smoked marijuana which I did not like. If I was going to get serious with him, I wanted him to know what I thought, however, I still wanted to go on another date with him. It was getting late so he drove me home and said he had a great time and would call me again.

A few days later he dropped by the house around 4:00 p.m. after work. I didn't expect it and I wasn't ready. I didn't feel like I was wearing the right clothes, just my grubby jeans and no makeup. Baba was home and saw him come over. I went outside and we sat on the front stoop. He held me by the waist and we talked and laughed. He kept staring at my eyes again, and that made me melt. He wanted to know if I would like to go over to his house sometime. So, one evening, he picked me up and drove to his house. We watched a new show on TV called, Different Strokes. He had his arm around me and said he liked the show, and I did as well. His little brother hung around and made little comments as we sat on the couch. Jesse finally had enough and told him to scram. I told him it was alright, but Jesse wanted to be alone with me. I also met his Dad who seemed to be indifferent toward me. I guess I wasn't the first girl Jesse brought home. It was a nice evening overall. I was starting to feel more at ease and I really enjoyed his company.

As he drove me home, I wondered if he would ask me out again, and then talked about the kind of music I liked. Taking things a step further, I told him there was an REO Speedwagon concert coming up and how it would be great to go on a double date with another couple. Abby couldn't go so I asked my cousin Ava. She wanted to go but didn't have a date. I told her to bring her brother as a favor to me, and I told Jesse my cousins would be coming with us. It was an outdoor concert, which was a first for me. I was really impressed, and I felt special. We had lawn seats all the way at the top where Jesse held me and gave me little kisses during the concert. My cousins were nearby and then I didn't see where they went. While we were kissing, one of Jesse's friends approached us and he quickly sat upright. His friend asked him if he wanted a "hit". I told Jesse I didn't approve, and he said no. His friend said, "since when"? Jesse told him he was cutting down and his friend started laughing and said, "I don't believe you man! You never say no". At this point I figured out what Jesse was really about. He did do drugs, however, I was impressed that he said no in front of me. Was he really doing that for me? I couldn't discount him now. Maybe he thought my opinion was valuable, and he did really like me as much as I liked him. Maybe I would be able to keep him away from drugs. I really didn't want him to ruin his life - he didn't know what it was like to live in a body that didn't function right. I wanted to tell him I had diabetes, but I was afraid to lose him if I told him the truth.

Jesse came over again on a Saturday and got to know my mom a little better. He came over in what I called an embroidered hippy shirt. My mom was a bit shocked by his shirt, but she was polite and offered him food which he gladly accepted. After meeting him again, she seemed to like him and I told her that he was going to quit doing drugs. I was so excited and happy and I was always thinking of Jesse. As a consequence, I lost 10 pounds in 2 weeks which took me to 120 pounds. That was really trim for my frame and I was the envy of my friends. My blood sugars were always high due to the adrenaline and I was probably in mild ketoacidosis most of the time.

My mom asked if I told him about my diabetes. I told her no. "Lucy", she said, "that's wrong, what if something happens to you, he won't know what to do." I thought, my blood sugar is always running high, I won't faint. I didn't even care about diabetes now because I had Jesse to think about. Around that time, I recall running to the bathroom and urinating constantly and I thought it was from all the diet soda I'd been drinking lately.

Jesse and I went on another date after that, and on our way home we were listening to the radio. I started singing Mick Jagger's song titled, "Under My Thumb". Jesse kept very quiet and dropped me off at home. I knew something was wrong because he didn't even kiss me goodnight, but I didn't know what. I waited for him to call me again, but after a week, he didn't. I was dying inside. What happened? I asked Abby if her friend had his number. I called him several times, but he wasn't home.

After several tries, I finally got him on the phone. I asked him if he was okay and he said yes. I asked him what was wrong and why I hadn't heard from him. He told me he didn't like being told what to do. I said, "what do you mean?" He said he didn't like being under my thumb. He said I was singing that song like I meant it. I said, "Jesse I didn't mean anything by that, I was just singing along." He didn't believe me and he thought I was trying to change him. I felt as if someone had dropped an elephant and crushed me. He didn't want to talk anymore and said he had to go. I could not believe he ended it this way and I was very hurt. I thought about him every day for about a year. It took me a long time to heal and as a consequence, I hid under my shell, and was very cautious about dating anyone else. My mom saw how I suffered from the break up and said "don't worry about it, he was a drug addict." I agreed, but I still cared about him even though we only knew each other for a short time.

I was still trying to find a good doctor as I was too old for a pediatrician. My mom took me to a hospital that specialized in diabetes. They had educational classes there and my mom signed me up for them. At the time, insurance would not cover them so the cost was all out of pocket. My mom didn't care, she wanted me to get in control and hoped they'd give me a stricter diet that I would have to start following.

I met with a dietician that put me on a program to balance my diet with my medication. I had to eat three meals per day with two snacks in between. I wasn't too crazy about this and I wasn't even sure I would do it. I was still on only one injection per day. They also recommended a new doctor that was a specialist in diabetes. The thought of all this just made me want to scream because I was so tired of dealing with diabetes. I didn't want to follow a diet, but I knew it was important and I didn't want to disappoint my mom. She had been through so much with me.

The nurse scheduled me for a class so I could share what I was doing with others. I thought maybe I would meet someone my age and I wouldn't feel so alone. The class was in the evening and everyone introduced themselves and shared some of their story. Many of the attendees were over the age of 30, and many of them were newly diagnosed. I felt like the diabetes dinosaur in the room, even though I was the youngest one there. When I introduced myself and told them I'd had diabetes for 16 years, they could not believe it. Most of the new diabetics were Type 2 meaning their bodies still produced insulin, yet have difficulty using it effectively. As the nurse started talking about the cause of diabetes and the impact of high blood sugar, we were told to stay away from sugars and starches, and to always measure everything on a scale. We were also told to start using the Accu-Check meter even if we only used the strips to see where the blood sugar level was. 180 mg/dl was the maximum amount recommended after eating. The nurse informed us about a new test called the glyco-hemoglobin test which measured how high our blood sugar had been over a three-month period. We were to take this test every 90 days with a goal of a glycohemoglobin level lower than 8. This was a lot to take in. Now there was a test to check up on me!

As the nurse went around the room to see if we had questions, a heavyset Italian woman who was just diagnosed shrieked and said, "I can't follow this diet, I can't cut out pasta, I'm Italian!" She was very defiant. The nurse said if she didn't follow the diet she would eventually suffer complications that might include gangrene, loss of vision, loss of kidney function, heart disease, and all the horror stories I had heard over the years. I looked over at my mom, and she knew what I was thinking. The woman said "I'm not going to follow this diet, I'm not giving up pasta!" At least she was older and had enjoyed her food up until this point. I just kept quiet and wanted to leave the room. Many people who get diagnosed as adults have great difficulty changing their ways. My grandmother was the same way.

The nurse had given us the name of my new doctor. My mom scheduled an appointment with him. I didn't know anything about this doctor and I hoped he was nice. I was taken into a room and the nurse took my weight and blood pressure. She was a bit rude. I waited with my mom and observed that the floors had dirt in the corners and the bottom of the table had splats of blood on it. I was already feeling uneasy. The doctor walked into the room. He was an obese bald man and it was hard to determine his age. He did not smile and he was not friendly as he looked over my chart. My mom started telling him that we'd made this appointment because my pediatrician could no longer treat me. He asked me how much insulin I was taking and if I was checking my urine every day for sugar. He proceeded to tell me that he was tough on his diabetic patients and he expected them to have blood sugars between 80 and 100mg/dl. I was starting to shake. He sounded like a sergeant and I felt my hands getting cold. How in the world was I going to get my sugar to that level? He said "I want you to meet another patient of mine, she's sitting in the waiting room." I thought, what could this be about, does he want me to make friends with someone? A tall blue-eyed, short blonde-haired girl walked into the room and she was looking down at the floor. She looked just a few years older than me. The doctor said "This is Donna. She has had diabetes for several years now and has severe diabetic retinopathy. Donna did not pay attention to her diabetes and used to have a candy bar for lunch most of the time. She now is legally blind and lost her job because her vision was very important to her work." Donna looked like she was about to cry and appeared to be shaking. The doctor was scolding her for not taking care of her diabetes and looking at me, finished with "do you want to end up like that?" My anxiety level was off the chart. All I thought about was how sorry I felt for her and then thought, is this what's going to happen to me? The doctor then said, "I want you to see something else." I thought, now what, another diabetes disaster? He had his nurse bring in a collage of baby pictures. He then said, "do you know who all these babies are?" I said, "no, are they all diabetics?" He said, "no, they are all perfectly normal babies of diabetic mothers." The doctor said "I have treated all these diabetic mothers monitoring them closely so they could have a normal child and childbirth." In a sense I was elated and that was a pleasant surprise. This gave me hope I could still have children someday and this put a whole new perspective on my life now. I was going to try and follow my diet and better manage my blood sugar.

I went home and started to follow the diet carefully. It was rough, and I really wanted to cheat. I craved sugar, so I would allow myself one piece of candy and savor it in my mouth. That would be my treat for the day. My mom would remind me when to eat my snacks. I just couldn't get used to a snack after dinner, and such a small one, like a few Saltine crackers or half a cup of milk. I started drinking diet soda in order to satisfy my sweet tooth. I could drink all I wanted, as long as I didn't overdo my food and kept away from sugar. As my blood sugar stabilized, I started to gain a little weight.

At my next appointment, the nurse weighed me and took my blood pressure. The doctor came into the room and with a stern voice said, "you gained weight." I felt guilty and I thought I had done everything right. I went from 125 pounds to 127 pounds. I didn't think it was a big deal. I wanted to be skinny enough to be attractive, just like any girl my age. He told me I needed to get those pounds off. I felt discouraged as I thought I was doing well by sticking to my diet.

I went home and continued the plan, trying not to eat as much. I was drinking more diet soda, but I didn't think that would make me gain weight, especially since it was diet.

I didn't even cheat with one piece of candy and I thought this time I would do better.

At my next appointment I wasn't happy to see him, but I needed my prescriptions. This time I wore shorts instead of heavy jeans, hoping that would show a better number. I was weighed again, and my blood pressure was taken. The doctor started pounding me about the weight, and told me I actually had gained another pound and that there was sugar in my urine. He continued to be harsh telling me that I was going to have complications if I didn't shape up. He said, "remember Donna? Do you want that to happen to you?" He said "I want to see you in two weeks and your results need to be better." I was miserable and near tears.

As we walked out of the office and down the hallway, I was scared for my life. I got in the car, and immediately broke out into a wailing cry. My mom said, "that's it, I'm not taking you back to him again." My heart was going crazy so I needed to calm down. She took me shopping to get my mind off of the visit and bought me a top that I liked. I still have it to this day. Despite leaving that doctor, his approach made me more afraid than ever about diabetic complications. Using Donna as a negative example made an impact on me but was simply abusive to her and should never be done.

I returned to school and enrolled in the Medical Assistant program which prepared students to work in a doctor's practice. It really wasn't my first choice, but I needed to finish college within one year. My new classes included typing and nursing classes, which were more clinical hands-on. In the back of my mind I was still reeling over the fact that I could not continue on as a Medical Lab Technician. I had to take Biology again, and I had to pass. I learned the same basic things over again and I passed with an A.

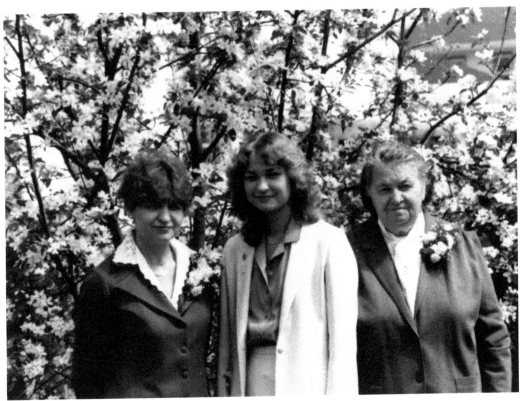

Mama, Lucy and Baba 1982

The second semester was more hands on and we learned more about nursing. We were taught how to apply bandages, deal with fractures, give immunizations, draw blood and give injections, take vital signs, give CPR, do simple office lab tests, dispose of contagious waste, sterilize instruments, and learned the basics of medical ethics.

In one of the classes, the instructor was going to teach us how to give injections using sterile saline solution. Injections was an area I knew all too well. I asked the instructor if I could talk to her about skipping injections on myself. The instructor agreed and the next day in class she told the class that I would be excused, because I already knew how to give injections due to the diabetes. I was relieved. I watched the other students' faces as they were giving themselves injections. There was sheer agony on some, bead of sweat on the foreheads of others, not to mention some shaky hands as they put the needle in their skin. I couldn't help but think now you people know how I feel every single day, sometimes more than once. Ha! You're getting a taste of my medicine. I will never forget that class and their reactions, but how could they possibly have understood how it was to live with injections on a daily basis, constantly hurting yourself and having to live with it? I was the only one that knew and it wasn't something I was proud of.

We had to complete a 6-week internship with a doctor's office as a part of our program's requirements. I was assigned to a family practice, where I would get experience working directly with patients. I got to practice checking patients in, doing vital signs, drawing blood, doing EKG's, writing prescriptions, giving injections and assisting with exams. The doctor thought I did great work and at the end of the internship, he asked if I could help out on Saturday mornings in his practice for five dollars an hour. I thought it was great to make some extra cash.

During the semester, we also had an ophthalmologist come to do a lecture about vision and eye health. As an eye specialist, he reviewed the subject of retinopathy and its complications. Fantastic! Now I can listen to complications of diabetic retinopathy. I almost skipped the lecture but reconsidered as this was information relevant to my condition. The doctor explained the various parts of the eye, the cornea, lens, vitreous humor and the retina. Then he started talking about what might cause retinopathy and of course, diabetes came up. I was hoping he would not call on me for anything. He did mention that diabetes was a factor for retinopathy, and that he was performing a new procedure in his office with a laser camera that could address the problem. Okay, I thought, interesting procedure, but does it really work and does it last?

I wondered if I had made the right decision becoming a Medical Assistant because I would always be faced with things that related to diabetes, something I tried to forget even though I had lived with it for 19 years. I stayed in the program, passed all the courses and took my final exam. I would be licensed and certified as a Medical Assistant; Lucy Krasno, CMA.

It was 1983, and graduation day had arrived. The family came to the ceremony and it was a proud moment for me. I was glad I made it that far.

After graduation, I took the summer to look for a full-time job as a Medical Assistant. I looked at postings at the college and I applied to a physician's office that was starting a new practice. I went to the interview and met all the doctors. They were all young, post-graduates. I enjoyed the interview and I was hoping to get the job. After a week or so, they called me and told me they had intended to offer me the job, but then decided to offer it to another student from my same class instead. I sulked. This couldn't have happened to me. Argh! Naturally, I reached for my go-to when I was stressed, something sweet to eat. I thought I deserved it.

I started looking in the newspaper every day for a job and I couldn't find any Medical Assistant jobs with physician practices. After a few weeks, I found a position for a Chiropractic Assistant. I applied, went to the interview and I got hired. I gained a lot of knowledge about the human body including chiropractic adjustments, supplements, hair analysis, traction and other holistic approaches. I was also able to participate in their screenings at no cost and I was intrigued to learn the results of my testing. The results came and I was told I was low in several things, such as sodium, magnesium, manganese and iron. My body made a lot of red blood cells, but they were tiny and I was low in hemoglobin, the oxygen carrying component of the blood. I was experiencing high blood sugar at that stage in my life with readings often over 200 mg/dl, and occasionally a healthier reading of 80 mg/dl. I also had an X-ray done on my back and was told I had a mild case of scoliosis.

The chiropractor put me on a number of supplements, which included magnesium, manganese, a certain pancreatic enzyme and a low dose iron supplement. I took these religiously for over a month, and then got retested. After I received the results I could not believe that all the deficiencies were in normal range. My blood sugar level remained high, although it was closer to 180 mg/dl.

I stayed on the supplements for a while, but it became too expensive to continue on my small salary. I thought maybe now that things were normalized, maybe they were fixed. I continued to take magnesium as a deficiency could contribute to muscle twitches I still had.

I started to get comfortable with my new job, taking case histories of new patients, administering ultrasound and traction, using EMG pads for muscle stimulation, applying hot packs and preparing paraffin baths for arthritis. I was very busy and was on my feet most of the day. Even though I was constantly moving, my blood sugar rarely went low or was life threatening. I felt more normal. I made friends with most of the assistants, except for the office manager who kept her distance.

My mom was thinking about finally buying her own place. Baba could live with my mom's brothers so she would not be alone. In 1983 we moved into a small two-bedroom condo, a short drive from Baba's house. Baba was disappointed by this change, and I would miss seeing her every day. Although somewhat daunting, it was good for me in that I had to become more independent and responsible for taking care of the house and adjusting to being alone more. I even bought some diabetic cookbooks with all the food exchanges listed. It was easy to follow and measure, and it helped me stay in better control. My mom and I redecorated the condo and it was fun.

I was now an adult with a responsible job and was also partly responsible for a home, and a car payment, paying for gas and oil changes. It was quite a change for me and it was a lot to get used to. I tried to never miss any days at work. I liked making my own money and being able to spend it. I was also very responsible and tried to save money when I could. I was able to stay on my mom's medical insurance until I was 22. Up until then, I never had to worry about paying much for insulin or syringes and thyroid medication. I tried to stay away from sugary foods as much as I could but it was always a challenge at the office at Christmastime or when there were birthdays. Cake, cookies or donuts were always there and I was embarrassed to say I couldn't eat them, so I would have a small piece just so I could fit in. They almost never had diet soda so I would always be stuck with water. Soon, Diet Coke came out on the market. Up until that time, Tab was the only diet soda I could drink. It was so great to finally be able to have a "Coke". I started to drink it almost every day - it was one of my simple pleasures. I also bought the latest Accu-Chek blood glucose meter. Diabetes is an expensive condition to have and I knew insurance coverage was important. The office where I worked did not cover employees with pre-existing conditions, so I was glad I could remain on my mom's plan for a while.

Our new neighbors decided to have a yard sale and I sat outside in the sun for the afternoon where I got a very mild sunburn. In a few days when my skin started to turn brown, I noticed a few areas where the burn wasn't resolving. It took a couple extra days for some areas on my neck, arms and around my eyes to disappear, and when they did, it left distinct white patches. It looked very unsightly, especially on my face. Why did I have these things on my skin? I remembered back when I was twelve and a little white patch had appeared on my left shoulder. I wondered if it was the same thing.

I showed my mom and then made an appointment with a dermatologist for the following week. He said it looked like one of two types of skin conditions; tinea versicolor or vitiligo. The first was caused by infection and the second had no known cause. He took a small skin scraping and sent it to the lab. I asked if there was treatment for either one of them and he assured me there was. As I returned to the office for my results, I was feeling really nervous. My skin test results showed that I had vitiligo and that this condition could spread all over my body. I was devastated. On top of diabetes, now this. I was in my early twenties, had just started my career and now would be hiding under long sleeves and avoiding dating.

The dermatologist said there was a treatment which involved taking a prescription and lying in a tanning bed several times a week. However, he wanted to try a tar solution on the areas first which smelled horrible. I came back in several weeks and told him it wasn't working. We moved to plan B where he prescribed a small pink pill to take one hour prior to every 30-minute session in the tanning bed.

He said this would take several treatments and last six months to a year. I purchased a $200/week tanning package which in addition to the cost of the medication consumed most of my paychecks. I went to the tanning salon about three times a week after work. I had to wear dark glasses after the treatment for about an hour so that I would not develop cataracts, which could be a side effect of the medication. I was a basket case thinking about this condition, trying to control diabetes and going to work pretending to be cheerful and acting like everything was okay.

After a month of these treatments, I was seeing some results. My skin pigment was coming back a little at a time. When I saw the dermatologist again, he was pleased with the results. He told me I could continue with the protocol, but could not say whether my skin would ever completely return to normal. I wondered if something in my new home caused this, but knew from the doctor that there was no known cause. Was this due to more stress from the recent changes in my life? I was determined to get rid of this and I completed the entire protocol. I looked for ways to cover the area around my eyes to conceal the white areas. I started wearing heavy eye shadow and mascara because I thought it would make me look a little more attractive. I seemed to still be attracting some guys.

Then out of the blue, a friend from my internship job called me and said there was a sales rep that wanted to get a group together to go bowling. He had taken a liking to me when I worked there. Evidently, he had expressed interest in me and was going to try and ask me out. I was embarrassed to date anyone now with this skin problem. I told my mom and she said, "just go!" Moms seemed to know best, so I hesitantly agreed to go bowling. It turned out to be a good time and Matt asked me for my phone number. I said okay, however, I don't think I knew what I was doing at the time. I figured I could just go and hide my skin problem, just like I had with the diabetes.

I made arrangements with Matt over the phone to go on our first date to an expensive restaurant downtown. When he told me where we were going, I just *had* to buy a new expensive dress to go there.

Matt arrived at the door looking like a million bucks with an expensive suit and tie. His car was immaculately clean. I almost felt like a princess as he opened the car door for me. He immediately started talking about himself, how he sold medical supplies during the day and worked part-time during the evenings and on weekends as an on-call firefighter. I was really impressed with him. I felt so small. I felt I had nothing to offer - I was just a diabetic with a weird skin condition. Why in the world would he want to go out with me? We arrived downtown at the John Hancock Center and the restaurant was on the 90th floor of the building. He put his arm out for me to hold onto and we walked in. The host took us to a window seat and we had the most spectacular view of the city at night – we could see for miles. I noticed the prices on the menu and I wanted to faint. I asked him what I should order, and he said whatever you want. Of course, I couldn't order *whatever* I wanted because there was this little thing called diabetes. I ordered the NY strip steak and mashed potatoes and Matt ordered the same dish. Matt was a gentleman all the way and I tried to be very lady-like. We didn't talk much, just smiled a lot. He didn't ask me too many questions which I liked because - I didn't want to reveal my dismal medical conditions.

For a moment I didn't even think about it. I was just in awe of his presence. I was being treated like a princess and it was the best feeling. I wasn't exactly sure if I liked Matt or not, but for this evening, it was a nice date. When we were done eating, I glanced at the bill and it was over a hundred dollars. This was a lot of money - it took me two days to make that much. After we left the restaurant Matt wanted to take me on a carriage ride through the city. Wow, what did I do to deserve this? We got in and Matt grabbed my hand. I was still feeling embarrassed and shy and I think he felt the same. I was smiling from ear to ear because it was a very special evening for me. On Monday, Matt sent me two dozen red roses at work, and all the girls at work were so impressed. They seemed a little jealous, so I felt a little uncomfortable. That date had been the most special date I'd ever had.

I received a wedding invitation from a family friend. My mom said, "why don't you ask Matt?" When I asked him to go with me to the reception, he was hesitant, but said okay. He told me he hated weddings. This was the first time I saw the other side of him. How could anyone who treated a girl like a princess, not want to go with her to a wedding reception for a few hours? I thought we would at least have some fun dancing.

It was the day of the wedding and I could tell Matt was not happy about it when he picked me up for the reception. I didn't like his comment about weddings, and thought maybe this was his way of saying he didn't want to get married. We arrived and I introduced Matt to Baba. Initially, she seemed to think Matt was a good match for me. He was dressed in a nice, expensive suit, and I wore a sparkly dress. Dinner was served, the band started to play and it was time for the first dance. I was hoping Matt would dance with me, but he had the biggest frown on his face. He was looking into space and paid no attention to me at all. I was trying to make conversation, but he barely spoke which upset me and was very disappointing. Baba pointed to the dance floor and nudged Matt to dance with me - he shook his head no. When Matt went to the men's room, Baba asked me why he was acting like he was at a funeral. I said "I don't know, but I'm not happy about it." When he came back, he asked me how much longer I wanted to stay. I said for a little while longer, I was hoping to dance at least one time. After the wedding was over, I was steaming. After having what had been the best first date, this date was horrible. The next time he called me, he told me that he didn't want to get married. I thought, fine I'm not going to marry you anyway.

Despite this, I continued to go out with Matt to the movies, bowling, to the mall, or just for something to do. As we walked in the mall one day, he kept looking at his hair whenever he passed a mirror. I said, "you look fine Matt". He said, call me "sir". After that he stopped calling me on the weekends to go out. He'd been busy working on his cars and firefighting, and evidently had no time to date or call me. I wondered if he was seeing someone else. At first, I didn't care, but actually, I felt hurt. After what would be our final date, he said "I'll call you." I made sure that was the end and decided it was best to focus on my job.

In 1984, I truly wanted to work in a regular medical practice. I applied to several medical practices and a podiatry practice that had called me for an interview ended up hiring me full-time. I began to work with computers, and assisting with patients. I also learned how to take off casts, take x-rays of the feet, change bandages and prep for minor surgeries. I was always worried about my blood sugars and eating lunch on time. I had to hide the white patches on my face and hands with a special stain I got from the pharmacy because I felt it made me look more presentable to patients.

I really hadn't encountered any patients with diabetic foot problems, but I always wondered about it. One day I had to cut a leg cast off of a patient with a special saw. It was getting close to lunch time and I had to make sure I wasn't having low blood sugar, so I ate some candy. One of the nurses was there watching me and noticed that I was very scared just holding the saw. I proceeded to start cutting from the knee to the ankle and the noise was disturbing. The nurse assured me that the saw would not cut the skin. I made it to the end of the foot and then had to pull the cast away from the gauze underneath. The patient said he was happy to get the cast off and I said "yes, me too!" I knew I was probably having high blood sugar at this point both from the adrenaline rush and the candy I had eaten. I tested my blood sugar and sure enough it was 240mg/dl, which definitely meant I was in ketoacidosis. I ate lunch and continued with the day. Many times I would operate like this, trying not to go low around patients.

After a year I moved on. I was hired at a general practice and worked for three different doctors and an obstetrician. They rotated every day, so I had to learn each of their styles. This was a brand new satellite office and I ran the whole office by myself, front and back. I made appointments, answered phones, checked patients in and out for their visits, filed, prepped patients for exams, took vital signs, drew blood and took EKG's. My responsibilities were very similar to what a nurse would do. One day, a patient referred from the hospital came in whose lower leg and foot had turned black from diabetes. He was an elderly man in a wheelchair and he was in pain and agony. I suddenly felt cold inside and wondered if this would be me in the future. I found out the man had a complicated medical history and was a smoker. After his exam the doctor came out of the room with me and said that his leg would need to be amputated. We told the patient his lower leg would have to be amputated to prevent the gangrene from spreading. If it continued to spread, he could die. My heart was with him. I could only imagine what he was going through. What a terrible consequence of diabetes. I tried hard to avoid thinking of myself in that situation. The patient came into the office for a follow up after his surgery. I remember being in awe because in addition to looking much better, he actually had a smile on his face. I felt so sad that he had to lose his leg to the monster called diabetes. He would be in a wheelchair for the rest of his life. Another life ruined by diabetes.

As I worked in this practice, I came in contact with other diabetic patients who I subtly gave preferential treatment to because I empathized with their situation.

I enjoyed working for the practice, but it was fast-paced and arduous. The 11-hour days on my feet were getting to be a bit too much. I was having a hard time managing my diabetes and paying proper attention to myself. My blood sugar was always running higher due to excessive fear of passing out in front of patients. This also contributed to a horrendous number of yeast infections which I would treat only to have it return.

The practice was very busy seeing an average of 40 patients per day. As the doctors signed more contracts with HMO's, the practice got busier and busier and the phone rang off the hook. My job became more and more demanding.

It was April of 1986 and my best friend Beth from junior high was getting married and she asked me to be her maid of honor. I was so happy for her because I knew how tough it was to find someone special. She asked me to help pick out the bridesmaid's dresses and luckily, we selected a dress that covered the vitiligo on my back, but I would still have to cover my arms with the stain.

Beth and her groom had a beautiful ceremony and I was really looking forward to the reception. I had stood up with Beth's brother Carl, who was very nice. I joked around with Beth's uncle who had taken me to senior prom. He put a cold glass filled with ice on my bare back while I was standing near the bar - I knew he was just teasing me. As I walked around the dance floor with another bridesmaid named Laurie, there were two young men who asked us to dance. They guy who asked me was very tall with blonde hair and green eyes. I thought he was attractive and I found out we had gone to high school together. He was a music teacher now and I found out he had just broken up with a long-term girlfriend he'd met in college. Beth and her new husband cut the wedding cake and, of course, I had a piece. Who cared how high my blood sugar was!

After the reception, Carl and a bunch of his friends asked me to join them with the other bridesmaids at a local bar for some more drinks and dancing. They were playing Madonna songs and we all sat around and talked. They all ordered alcoholic drinks, mostly beers, but I ordered a diet coke. My dance partner questioned why I didn't order a cocktail, and I just flat out told him I didn't drink. He asked me to slow dance a few times and seemed interested in me. It was getting toward 3:00 a.m. and he asked me for my phone number, so I told him he could get it from Beth. A few days went by and I called Beth's mom to have her tell him that it was okay to call me. I felt like a fool. My mom said, "why didn't you just give him your phone number in the first place?" I knew why – I didn't want to get involved with someone knowing my diabetes would get in the way. I would have to explain my diet, my blood sugar testing, long-term effects on the body, vitiligo, hypothyroidism and God knows what else. I was sure he would reject all of it. Despite all of that I still took a chance. A few days went by and Brad called me. I was excited because I didn't expect the call, but I kept it cool on the phone. He didn't seem too enthusiastic at first, but after we talked for a while, he asked me to go out for pizza, which is not a great choice for diabetics. I could feel my blood sugar rising just thinking about it. As we talked, he asked me what I like to do outdoors. I told him bike riding and he said, "I love bike riding!" From that point we hit it off. He liked to joke around, and I liked to laugh at his jokes. Though we'd gone to high school together, for the life of me, I couldn't remember who he was until I looked him up in my yearbook. After our first date, he dropped me off at home and didn't kiss me at the door so I thought he was rejecting me. I went inside and went right to sleep. My blood sugar was high from the pizza.

Brad called me again and this time we went out to an amusement park. More dates followed —we rode bikes, went dancing, and did other fun things. Brad was a refreshing change to my life. With all the demands of my job and diabetes, being with Brad took my mind off all my problems. I enjoyed spending time with him and going to parties with mutual friends. There was never a dull moment with Brad. We had dated for six months and I hadn't told him I was a diabetic, I was having such a good time, why spoil something good? I didn't know that Carl, Beth's brother, had already told him I had diabetes. Despite dating for six months, Brad had never said "I love you". One evening, when we were alone in a quiet moment, I had asked him (motioning to myself), "do you love this girl?" He replied back, "yes, yes I do. I love you", he said. I had awakened the sleeping giant. Love it was! I told him I loved him back. We officially belonged to each other.

Brad then told me that he knew I had diabetes. At first he didn't believe Carl. He would even look for medications in my refrigerator when I wasn't there but never found any. I kept my insulin vials in a case where they were not immediately visible. Brad used to work in a pharmacy when he was in high school and he knew what he was looking for. He asked me if Carl was right. I looked down at the floor and I said "yes, it's true." I almost wanted to cry and hoped he wouldn't leave me. Brad said he'd known for a while and was amazed that he never saw me treat my diabetes. It was difficult to continue hiding and now it was finally out in the open. I felt an enormous burden was lifted from my shoulders. He told me it was okay, and that he still loved me for me. Finally, I could show him my medications and let him know what diabetes was really about.

Chapter Five

<hr/>

HAPPILY EVER AFTER?

BRAD AND I continued seeing each other for two years. This was the longest relationship I had experienced, and I began to wonder if he loved me enough for marriage. I was 27 years old, and I never once heard Brad talk about marriage. Was he stringing me along, just to have someone on his arm? I started to get a little angry. It had been two years since Beth got married and she already had a baby. My diabetes wasn't getting any better and I had to think about having children and how the longer I waited, the greater the risk factors for carrying a baby. I told my mom if Brad didn't make a move soon to get married, I was going to break it off with him. She told me, "oh no, don't do that, he really loves you and cares, don't give up on him." She was right, he already knew about my condition. I would have to start all over with someone else and go through this again. I didn't want to do it so I continued to see Brad. Besides, Valentine's day was coming up. Just another card and a box of candy I can't have, I thought.

It was February 1988 and Brad was going to take me downtown to see the symphony orchestra. He was planning to wear a tuxedo and I was thrilled to go shopping to buy the perfect dress for the occasion. As I walked into a local specialty store, they were unloading dresses off of a rack. I saw the perfect dress – it was bright red with a big bow in the back and rhinestones in the middle of the bow. It fit perfectly and made me look elegant and feel wonderful. It hid all my skin imperfections.

On the evening of February 13, Brad arrived at the door wearing a tux, looking handsome, with his blonde hair slicked back. He wore a red bow tie to match my dress and we looked so great as a couple. He gave me a corsage to wear and my mom took several photos of us and some of just me in the dress. I thought, why all this fuss?

We arrived at a famous restaurant in downtown Chicago that ironically, had opened its doors on Valentine's Day in 1898. The waiter immediately took a liking to how my open-back dress looked. Brad said, "look but don't touch!" I just smiled. We ordered prime rib, mashed potatoes and a dessert that we shared. Diabetes wasn't even in the picture. It was so romantic! While we were eating, an older woman came by our table and said "Congratulations dear!" I was confused, why would she say that? After the meal, Brad said he had something for me. He swiftly took a little black box out of his coat pocket and put the box on the table. As he opened the box, there was a beautiful diamond ring inside and he asked me if I would marry him. I looked at it and him and started to tear up. I took the box and nervously closed it. I said "yes, I will marry you." He opened the box and slipped the ring on my finger. We were officially engaged, and I was happy but apprehensive at the same time. Brad walked proudly out of the restaurant with his head held high with my arm on his, as we walked down the street to his car.

We arrived at Orchestra Hall and it was vast. Brad planned well because we had top row seats in the middle facing the orchestra. This brought back memories of my grade school field trip. As a music teacher Brad was in awe. I enjoyed the performance, but my heart was racing. I couldn't figure out if it was due to my blood sugar being high or just the excitement of the event. I kept looking at the beautiful diamond ring as I held Brad's hand.

Brad drove me home and we hugged and smiled at each other. I walked through the door and my mom was waiting up for me. I said, "you're still up?" She said, "Congratulations!" She said she had known about this for several weeks already because Brad had asked my mom for my hand in marriage. I said "both of you are sneaky!" Then I showed her my ring. She said "it's bigger that the one I got before I got married!" I was joyful, but at the same time uncertain. I suspected that was normal for anyone thinking about marriage for the first time. For me it was different. I had this thing called diabetes in the way, not to mention hypothyroidism and vitiligo. I wanted to have a family, but how would we handle it? I was uneasy throughout our engagement.

Brad and I went to visit Baba that following weekend to tell her the news and show her my engagement ring. Baba was happy and said "I'll wear a long, pink dress to your wedding," my favorite color.

Soon thereafter Baba began to feel unwell. She'd been suffering with severe back pain. She had also been dealing with diabetes for over 10 years and I wondered if it was her kidneys. Baba didn't manage her diabetes well and I told her to come in to the office where I worked for a checkup. The doctor took an x-ray of her back and discovered she had severe osteoporosis. Baba was also diagnosed with ALS and was given less than a year to live as there was no cure. I didn't think much of it at the time because I thought the doctor was wrong. This just can't be! Baba was a strong woman and she raised six children. The doctor had to be wrong. I made a copy of the doctors' notes and took them home for my own reference. As time passed, Baba became weaker and had to support herself first with a cane, then a walker. I was hoping she would make it to my wedding.

Brad and I started to spend every weekend planning our wedding. I had to find a dress, a venue, do wedding invitations, and select our wedding party. We had to buy wedding rings and decide where we wanted go for our honeymoon. We also needed to find an apartment.

Baba needed a lot of support and within a few months, she was seriously declining. It was the hottest summer we'd ever had and Baba could barely walk and had to be on oxygen 24 hours a day. She spent all her time indoors with air conditioning. By September, the doctor placed her in the ICU with a very bad case of pneumonia. She could no longer talk, and could only make small movements with her eyes and fingers. A thought came to my mind that said if she makes it past the 23rd, she will live, if not she will pass away. The 23rd, came and Baba made it through the day sitting up in bed and seeming to feel better. I was relieved and really thought she would make it out of the hospital. Baba remained alert for several weeks but her body was deteriorating. I was crying inside and knew we were losing her. I remember when the priest had come to pray over her, Baba was able to make a sign of the cross with her right hand on the bed as the priest was speaking. I prayed along with them, as did my mom.

Brad wanted me to go to a local town where they were celebrating Octoberfest. I wasn't in the mood because I knew my mom and uncles were taking turns going to the hospital, but I went anyway. Brad dropped me off at Baba's house around 11:30 p.m. As I walked in the house, a candle was lit on the table. Mom whimpered to me "she's not going to live". I laid down on the bed next to my mom and closed my eyes to try and relax. The phone rang and I knew it was bad news. The nurse called to say Baba passed away peacefully in her sleep. Mom and I started sobbing. I tried to pull myself together and called Brad to let him know what happened. In a sleepy voice he said, "Oh, I'm sorry Lucy". When we arrived at the hospital, I remember the room was still and all the life support machines were turned off. I looked at Baba (her skin turned yellow in color). I touched her and she was still warm. I bent over to kiss her on the forehead and said, "goodbye, I love you, I will always love you." Baba was so very important having cared for me almost from birth. I really thought she would live forever. A person I loved and could lean on was gone. As we all stood in the room to say our goodbyes, Brad walked in. He had driven up to the hospital out of love for me.

The following day was very sad and I dreaded going to the funeral home to make arrangements. As the curator drew up the paperwork, he wrote October 24th. My premonition was right. Baba didn't make it past the 23rd, it was just a month later. We picked out a large bouquet of red roses for the casket. I chose a special red rose and a pink corsage to go inside the casket (from me) to rest with Baba. We were all very somber at the wake. When we arrived at the funeral home to view the body my mom and I immediately started crying. We walked up to the casket and I put my hand on Baba's hand. It was ice cold. The warm hand that I held thorough out my childhood was now cold and lifeless. I could not grasp this reality and I was hoping the stress would not send me into ketoacidosis. This was the first time I lost a close family member that I loved and I remember praying in that moment that I wouldn't have a heart attack. I'd had diabetes for 24 years at that point and wondered why it wasn't me. How could I still be alive? I should have already died, but it wasn't my time. My mom, Baba and I could not have been closer and I had to stay strong for my mom.

The guests had started to arrive and the room was filled wall-to-wall with flowers. Brad sat next to me as the priest started the eulogy. He described Baba's life as she escaped WWII with the family from her beloved country of Ukraine. She had survived the bombings, the Soviet manmade hunger of 1933, moved to several unknown countries while her kids were young, and lost her husband to a bicycle accident in Brazil, leaving her to raise the children on her own, instilling in them the importance of knowing God and to always better themselves with an education. Baba had overcome so much in her life but in the final years faced the diabetes enemy as well.

The following day was the funeral and it was a very cold, blustery day. After the funeral service, the hearse drove her body past the house and then on to the cemetery. The priest said several prayers and they lowered the casket gently into the ground as family members wept. I threw a red rose on to the casket with others as they threw black dirt on the casket. It was so painful to know that Baba would never be at my wedding wearing said that long, pink dress she'd talked about. I walked away from the cemetery with Brad, sobbing while he held on to me.

Mom had gone back to work and so did I. We started to accept life without Baba and it was especially hard for my mom. We talked several times a day. There was a lot of adjusting to do, but everything would be okay.

As things started to settle, Brad and I continued to plan our wedding. His mom recommended where I could get a really nice yet inexpensive wedding dress. I had already tried on a few dresses and had always admired the off-the-shoulder dress that Princess Diana the Princess of Whales wore at her wedding in 1981. I tried on a similar dress, but my skin condition seemed to overtake the dress, so it was out of the question.

I tried on another dress that was beautiful. It wasn't my first choice, but because of the vitiligo I settled for it.

I had asked several friends to stand up in my wedding with Beth being my first choice for maid of honor since I had stood up in her wedding. Katy, my childhood friend was also asked.

As the months went by there were many details to take care of. Brad and I were not raised in the same religion. He was Catholic and I was Eastern Orthodox but Brad insisted on getting married in my church. The cemetery where Baba was laid to rest was near the church and it was comforting that she would be close-by. The church was beautiful with a golden dome and a cross on top. Shortly before the wedding, a conflict arose between Brad and his father. Apparently, his father wanted him to marry a Catholic girl. I felt it was Brad's responsibility to take care of this with his father. The difference in our religions didn't matter to me, I was just happy that someone loved and accepted me in spite of my health conditions. That was the only thing that mattered to me. As we continued with wedding plans, there was another conflict. I was happy with a DJ we'd selected for the reception, but Brad's father was insisting on a Polka band. Stress levels were rising. At one point, I told Brad I was not going to mail out the wedding invitations until this was resolved. Unfortunately, Brad's father got his way. Was I making the right decision? What if I never found someone else who would accept me with diabetes? I was tired of being with the wrong person. Brad watched me test my blood sugar and give myself injections and it didn't bother him. That verified my decision. Brad's love and continued support was enough evidence for me to see he wanted to be there. He told me "I'm going to push you around in a wheelchair when you're old and gray." He was in it for the long haul. In final preparation for our new life together, Brad and I went through Pre-Cana (Catholic marriage counseling) with the priest from his parish and it went very well.

The wedding weekend arrived and I had to work on Friday (the day of the rehearsal). After work, I picked up my youngest bridesmaid and drove with her to the rehearsal. After the rehearsal on Friday, we went to a local pizza restaurant and had dinner. I gave all the bridesmaids, amethyst and gold necklaces as a token of my thanks. They were very surprised by the gift of fine jewelry. By 10:00 p.m. I was tired and wanted to get some sleep before the big day. I was hoping Brad would drive home and follow behind me, but he wanted to stay at the restaurant so I said, "I'll see you tomorrow." I was upset as I drove home alone on the expressway. I walked in the door, my mom and my aunt Nadia were waiting for me. My mom asked, "are you by yourself?" I said "yes", very unhappily. She whispered, "he didn't come with you?" I said "no." Now my mom was upset too. She couldn't believe Brad would not follow me home before the wedding. I was not in very good spirits.

I woke up the next day, took my medication, had breakfast and went to the beauty salon to get my hair done for the wedding. It had rained in the morning and my hair was not holding up very well in the humidity. This was my special day and I didn't want anything to go wrong. I came back home and made sure I had enough to eat. I wasn't about to faint at my wedding! I put on my makeup and then proceeded to cover the white spots of vitiligo on my hands so the imperfections would not be seen in a lot of the photos. As I was putting on my wedding dress, my bridesmaids started to arrive. Surprisingly, I was not as nervous as I thought I would be. After the photos, the limo arrived and we drove off to the church. As we arrived, everyone was anxiously waiting to see the bride. In the Orthodox church, the bride and groom enter the church at the same time and after the priest does a short ceremony at the entrance, they follow the priest to the alter. Brad and I smiled as we saw each other. He said I looked beautiful and complimented my dress. The ceremony was an hour long followed by lots of pictures in the church. Diabetes didn't affect our ceremony and I was so happy I didn't faint!

Our reception went on for several hours with dancing, walking around to visit guests at the tables and cutting the cake. My legs were hurting because I had been on my feet practically all day. When we left for the evening, I told Brad to stop somewhere and buy me some aspirin. I said "if I don't have aspirin, I will not have a good night." My blood sugars were probably high all day. I never had a moment to check it.

Brad had surprised me after the ceremony with a hotel room that had a hot tub. I was exhausted from the day, and tried to be pleasant about the surprise. The diabetes was catching up with me. Brad had a better evening than I did. The following day, we were going to Hawaii. My Godfather had gifted us with tickets for the trip.

The wedding fairytale came to an end after we returned. I was now a married woman with more responsibilities. We moved into an apartment that was not too far from both our jobs. I still worked at the doctor's office and Brad worked in the city teaching high school music. The apartment was costly, but Brad wanted me to have a nice place to live. After a year in the apartment, my mom offered to let us live in her house at no cost so we could save money for a while. Mom would move in with my uncles to help them out now that Baba had passed away. Brad was not very happy with the situation from the beginning, but he agreed. At one point we got into an argument and he packed his suitcase to leave. I asked him to stay and talk things out and he reluctantly agreed. I wondered what I had gotten myself into. He said he was uncomfortable living in my mom's house and he wanted a house of his own. I agreed to the idea, but I wasn't sure what kind of home we would qualify for since neither of us had a large salary. Plus, a significant amount of money I earned went towards paying for insulin, syringes and thyroid medication.

We looked at homes we could afford, close to my mom's. We decided on a ranch house that was built in the 1960's. It was a very small house with an eat-in kitchen, living room and three bedrooms. We signed the mortgage and quickly moved in. We did not have a lot of items to move. The house did not have a washer and dryer so we needed to purchase them. In order to save money on a delivery fee, Brad said he could use his little brother's pickup truck to get them. When Brad's father realized the truck was gone from his driveway and that Brad had used it to move our new appliances, they got into a huge argument. It appeared that Brad's father was not interested in helping us and I began to notice that Brad never stood up for me in front of his father. I told him, "tell him I am your wife!" After he got off the phone, he said his father was reneging on the $5,000.00 he had promised to give us for remodeling. I felt his bias against me was tied to our religious differences.

Brad found a job closer to home but was hesitant because it was an elementary school. He ending up taking the position. Since he was changing positions, I asked him to put me on his health insurance policy since my own coverage was poor. Brad told me ultimately, he wanted to get a job where he could be a band director and talked about getting a Master's Degree. I wondered why he waited to get married before thinking about pursuing a Master of Music because it was going to cost time and money. He would have to take evening courses and he had told me he wanted to have a family of at least three children. I was troubled. After 24 years with diabetes would I even be able to have three children? Would there be complications? I kept disagreeing with the idea of three children and thought we should just try for one. I wanted to be financially stable before we started having a family. I asked him if he would be open to adoption and he said no. Soon, I started to see another aspect of his character emerge. After a while, Brad started to go out with his married buddies from high school and college. He was invited to a bachelor party for a close friend that was getting married and I didn't approve of it. He was married, and what were they doing at those bachelor parties? I knew there was going to be heavy drinking involved and Brad *loved* beer —I hadn't realized how much until after we got married. He had at least one beer every day after work and continued to hang around his buddies every opportunity he got. I was alone much of the time.

One evening, he decided he was going to meet one of his friends. I didn't know where he was going. It was past midnight and I kept looking at the clock. Where was he? I didn't want to call my mom and worry her unnecessarily. I had no way to contact him. Finally, around 2:00 a.m., I heard the door open and I pretended to be asleep. He got into bed and he reeked from alcohol. I couldn't sleep the rest of the night. I laid in bed with my eyes open. Brad fell asleep right away, he was completely drunk.

The following morning, I got out of bed as soon as the sun was up. Brad didn't get up until much later and when he woke up, I confronted him. He told me he needed to go drinking with one of his friends who lived 40 miles away. Immediately, I said "are you crazy? You drove home like that? What did you drink, you smelled really bad." He told me they were drinking vodka. I lost it. I said, "how could you drive home like that, you could have killed someone! Legally, they would most likely come after me if something happened to you". He said he needed to get away.

Brad and I started drifting apart and he never mentioned having a family anymore. When I would ask him, he didn't even want to talk about it. I made an appointment with my doctor to ask him where my blood sugars needed to be in order to have a baby. After two months I was able to get my A1C blood levels in the acceptable range to conceive. I came home excited and he didn't seem happy at all. He began to ignore me more and more and I felt so alone. I talked to my mom every day on the phone. When I told her what had happened she said, "don't even think about having children with him." I went over to her house and began to cry. I said, "what am I supposed to do? I am getting closer to 30 and it will not be easy to have children without the risk of more complications". She said, "I'm not going to meddle, but you know what happened with your father." I was suffering with the stress of our failing marriage, but I really didn't want a divorce.

The next time I spoke to Brad, I mentioned marriage counseling. I offered to pay for it, and he reluctantly agreed. When we saw the marriage counselor, she complemented us on what a cute couple we were, then her questions quickly caused an argument. She then said, "you make such a nice couple and I can't understand why there is so much tension between you." She gave us some exercises to do at home, but Brad never wanted to do them. We saw the counselor for a few weeks, and I could tell that Brad was checked out. He didn't think he was doing anything wrong in the marriage and the counseling didn't help.

We continued to drift further apart, and on the weekends he made his own plans and did whatever he wanted to without me. I still wanted to know his thoughts about starting a family. Maybe there was still a glimmer of hope. He finally told me "I decided two years ago I didn't want to have children with you." He might as well have stabbed me in the back. Divorce was the last thing I wanted, but I couldn't continue living with a liar. I knew my chances were now very slim to ever have children of my own. From that point on, I was living in an empty marriage. This went on for several months until I could save up enough money for a lawyer. I stopped making dinners and just fed myself – anything out of cans and microwave dinners. I found a lawyer I could see on my lunch hour and after a few weeks, the lawyer served Brad with divorce papers at his job. He came home and didn't say a word to me. He got up the next morning and left me a note that he was going out to take photos and didn't know when he would be back. I moved out of the house that day. It was a very sad ending to a marriage that I had expected to last a lifetime.

While I never got to know my father, I had inadvertently gone ahead and married someone very similar to him. If I was to be given another chance at marriage, I certainly would be more vigilant with my choice.

Chapter Six

Chapter Six

CAREER FOCUS

AFTER THE DIVORCE, I lost a lot of weight and tried to pick up the pieces of my broken life. I got a new job that offered benefits and health insurance through a friend of mine. I didn't want the stress of working for doctors anymore. The job was a longer commute for me, but the money was good. I moved back in with my mom who was now working for a school district doing payroll.

In 1992, the Soviet Union was breaking up and Ukraine, the homeland of my ancestors, was finally becoming free after 70 years of communism. My uncles started to travel to see family members there. My mom said, "I would love to go to Ukraine." I thought about my diabetes and my ability to travel there. The medical system there was third world and at this point, and after having diabetes (and its associated health issues) for 30 years, I was very reluctant. I agreed to go and decided I would need to bring double the amount of supplies of insulin, syringes, thyroid medication and blood sugar test strips. I also brought a prescription of broad-spectrum antibiotics just in case. My uncle Paul said he would pay for our flight and go with us for support. We booked the trip and planned to spend three weeks in Ukraine. It was a long time to be away from home, so I packed extra food and even brought some diet soda with me in my suitcase. I wasn't sure what they would serve us there, or how often we would have meals or water. It was a risk traveling there with diabetes, but it was so important to me to see where Baba came from and understand more about my roots.

After a nine-hour flight, we arrived in Kiev, Ukraine and we walked through a shabby looking airport. This is how I had imagined the Soviet Union would be. We stood in line to check in at the passport counter and there was a large glass screen with a clerk standing behind it and a mirror hanging off the ceiling. As I approached, the attendant spoke in a thick stern Russian accent saying "PASSPORT". I was terrified and felt very intimidated. After he compared me to my photo several times, he quickly gave my passport back. It was the coldest greeting I'd ever had and I couldn't help but wonder how the rest of the country would be.

We went to baggage claim, and everyone was speaking in Russian. My mom was appalled and said "why are you not speaking in Ukrainian?" They noticed an American flag on my suitcase so we were able to get through with all my diabetes supplies. I was relieved.

One of Baba's family members picked us up from the airport. We arrived at my mom's cousin Ida's house who lived in Kiev with her daughter. They lived on the top floor in an apartment complex and we had to carry our heavy suitcases up three floors. This was going to be a challenge. The apartment rooms were very small. They showed me my bed which was very lumpy and hard. I didn't expect this. Our family hosts would spend the night at their friend's, so we could use their beds. This was their way of showing hospitality to us. Ida would come back in the morning and cook breakfast for us. I didn't really know what I was eating or how much sugar it had in it. I just ate less, so I wouldn't have to think about it. When Ida wasn't there, I would take some potato chips out of my suitcase and eat them. Ida caught me and got very upset that I hardly ate what she made, and then ate those chips. I felt badly about that. I'd brought a six pack of diet Mountain Dew and had two per week so it would last the entire trip. In Ukraine, the only types of drinks that were available were mineral water (which tasted awful) or Coca-Cola – but only in the city. We left the apartment to see the city of Kiev. I brought a brand new camcorder to record the trip. While the foliage was beautiful, most of the buildings in the city were in dire need of repair. The shelves in most stores were nearly empty. I never saw such scarcity in my life. There were bread lines and it felt like what occurred in the Great Depression in the United States. Fear came over me. How was I going to survive here with diabetes? God help me, don't let me get sick. I felt a million miles from home.

We walked around the city of Kiev all day and luckily, we found a restaurant where I had some different foods to choose from. We had perogies and the portions were smaller as compared to what we were used to back home. We stayed at Ida's place for a week, and then took another flight to where Baba used to live with her family in a southern city in Ukraine called Poltava. This is the town where my mom was born.

We arrived in the village and about 30 family members were there to greet us. They were very excited and kissed us enthusiastically. Baba's sister was there, and I noticed she had the same hands and gestures, and a similar sense of humor. I thought a lot about Baba when I was there, and it was so special to see where she lived and started to raise her family. Baba's sister was in her 70's and I could just imagine how beautiful she must have been when she was younger. I also met two relatives in the village that were diabetics, clearly part of our family genetics. One man was already quite ill with an amputation and was bedridden. I could tell by his face that he was in agony and likely could not get adequate health care. As we visited, he just kept talking about his illness. I wasn't really interested in hearing too much about it. I felt empathy but there was nothing I could do to help him. This reminded me of how crippling and merciless diabetes could be. After another week in the village with an unpredictable diet and not getting enough sleep, I became ill myself. I was fearful and wondered what would happen if this was serious. Fortunately, the nausea and vomiting lasted one day before I felt better. My mom's cousin Helen helped to take care of me and I was so happy that it turned out to be a 24-hour bug or reaction to something I ate.

The children in the village gave me a tour which included the outhouse as they had no indoor plumbing at all in their home. The family's kitchen was actually in a separate building apart from the house. There was a huge farm, where they grew as much as possible and canned everything in order to survive in the winter. I just imagined how hard their lives were. I was so grateful I had the medical care I needed and felt very lucky to live in America. I saw the home that Baba lived in and I felt a connection to her just being there. Those family members really made me feel like I was at home. I enjoyed staying in the village and they had more food than I expected. There was always a meat, carbohydrate and vegetable item at every meal and Helen and her daughter were wonderful cooks. They made the food look so appetizing, even though there were minimal cooking utensils to help them. The teenagers in the village were in awe of the diet Mountain Dew I had, and I wish I had brought more to share with them.

My mom came down with a severe sinus infection when we were there and ended up using my antibiotics to treat it. I was praying I wouldn't need them for the rest of the trip.

After a week in the village, we took an overnight train ride to another town in the north called Ternopol to visit another one of my mom's cousins. We traveled on an old-style Soviet Union train sleeper car with four cots that had to be shared with strangers. The train stopped at various stations and they blew the loud horn at every stop all night long. None of us got any restful sleep.

We finally arrived at Ternopol and met my mom's other cousin Helen. She lived in a nicer, more spacious apartment in the city. On the wall was an embroidered picture of Vladimir Lenin (Russian Communist leader). My mom confronted her about why she had this hanging on her wall. She said it was one of the treasures she embroidered. I began to see what influence the Soviet Union KGB had on the Ukrainian people and how so many years later Lenin's face was still precious to her. Helen had a shower in her apartment and I couldn't wait to use it. The government completely shuts off the water for seven hours every day and if you don't take a shower in a certain time frame, you miss the opportunity. I couldn't believe there was so much control over people's lives.

Mom and I visited with Helen in her town and even met some of her friends. Some of them had a few more "luxuries", like a refrigerator and fresh linens for the bed. As I understood it, they had some nicer things because they either had ties with the government or they knew someone from the United States who was helping them out. I finally took a shower after a week and was able to curl my hair. I couldn't believe I was able to manage my diabetes in Ukraine. I was getting exercise from all the walking around, which must have kept my diabetes in check.

We decided to visit the beautiful Carpathian Mountains. We spent a day there and as we entered the forest, I recall it seemed really barren. I didn't see any wildlife, not one bird or insect. I wondered if this was the impact of the nuclear explosion in Chernobyl in 1986. Helen said people did come there to hunt for animals and food. We hiked up a mountain that had small concrete steps that took us high enough where the beauty of the mountainside could be seen. I enjoyed the beautiful mountains, clean air and took in the breathtaking views. This was one of the highlights of the trip. We spent the remainder of the week with Helen and explored her town, but soon it was time to go home.

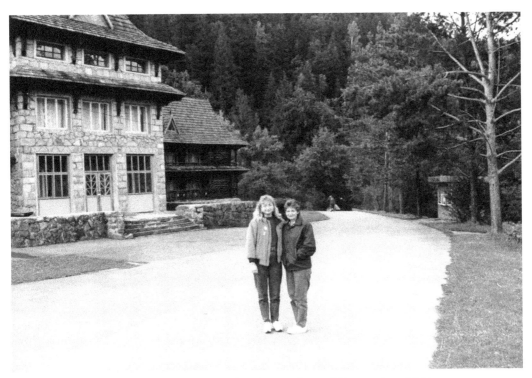

Lucy and Mama in the Carpathian Mountains 1993

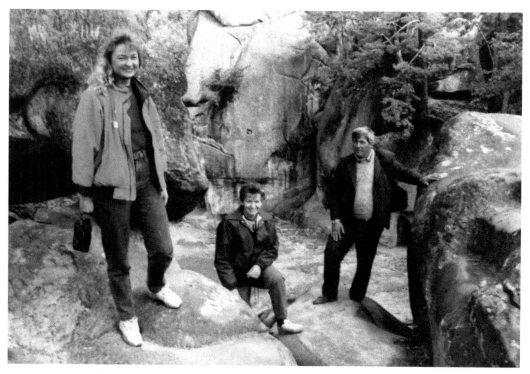

Lucy, Mama and relative on mountaintop in Ukraine

We connected through France on the way back home. When we arrived, we immediately went to a restaurant to have dinner and the waiter brought us extra fruit and rolls. We ate everything because we were so hungry for "normal" food. The waiter was flabbergasted that everything on the table was gone before our dinners were served. We were never so happy to eat! I had lost 10 pounds in the three weeks we spent in Ukraine. Though I enjoyed it, I was ready to come home. The flight was long and when we arrived in the States, I was thankful we made it home safely and wanted to kiss the ground. Again, I was lucky to live in America – where freedom rings.

I returned back to work in a new position, I was working with computers doing inventory control on an IBM DOS system which dated back to the 1980's. I had to learn from scratch. It was a basic black screen with bright green letters on it. I enjoyed doing the work. The money was very good, but I needed to wait 90 days until I qualified for health insurance benefits. Working for and being covered under a larger corporation's health care plan, I knew I wouldn't experience discrimination for having pre-existing conditions. Before I was married, health insurance and costs associated with diabetes took a significant portion of my paycheck every week. Diabetes care is expensive.

In the office things were getting complicated. My boss's supervisor got romantically involved with the friend who got me the job. Subsequently, the supervisor was fired and because of my connection to the situation through my friend, I was let go as well. The situation had nothing to do with my job performance. I was devastated to have lost all my benefits and start looking for another job.

Soon after this I came down with a very bad upper respiratory infection. My immune system was further compromised due to the stress of losing my job. My doctor put me on a two-week regimen of antibiotics, but it did not clear up. I continued to get worse and developed a very bad case of bronchitis. Even after two weeks of bed rest, I still had the cough. I visited my doctor's office again and the doctor put me on more antibiotics. Unfortunately, this triggered another yeast infection and I also began to wheeze. My mom was really concerned so she said, "lets drive to Florida for a week, you could be in the sun and get some warmth, maybe that will take care of the infection." However, I knew my vitiligo was going to make it difficult for me to be in the sun. The hotel we stayed in was near a mineral springs pond. A woman who worked there was a naturopath, and my mom told her we were there to get some warmth so I could recover from my bronchitis. This woman knew a lot about unconventional treatments and she mentioned that taking a combination of Goldenseal and Echinacea herbs strengthens the immune system and would help me to get rid of the bronchitis. She gave me some samples and I began taking them, and experienced no side effects. She had also told me to stop taking them after two weeks (or sooner if I felt better before then). After returning home and locating what I needed at a health food store, I took the herb for three days and my infection was gone. I was astonished and I felt so much better! At this time, I also decided to try a vegetarian diet that included beans and rice, and fruits and vegetables. In other words, I had to give up meat, poultry and eggs. Due to the heavy amount of carbohydrates I was now ingesting, I needed to give myself extra injections of fast acting insulin at meal time. My blood sugar seemed to spike more often due to all the starchy foods and this led to an increase in my glyco-hemoglobin A1C levels and yes, more yeast infections. My doctor was not happy with me. I knew from studying diabetes that too much protein in the diet can affect the kidney function, so I started eating protein again but just in smaller portions.

Now that I had finally recovered, I began to look aggressively for a full-time job.

I attended job fair in order to get my resume out to more employers. I put on a professional-looking suit, with shoes and purse to match and brought 25 copies of my resume. I left my resume at many of the booths and a temporary agency was very interested in background. They asked if I knew of any of the new Microsoft applications (Word, Excel, PowerPoint) or Word Perfect. I said I didn't, but I had experience using computers for manufacturing and inventory control. The following day, the agency called me to say they had an opening for a temporary job at a company that manufactures and services tool and die machinery. The money was a few thousand less per year than my last position, but I took the job because I needed it.

When I started the new job, I didn't tell anyone I had diabetes and I worked hard to manage it so that I wouldn't have low blood sugar in the office. In the process, I got addicted to diet Mountain Dew and was drinking three to four cans per day. I still ate my normal meals but I was also eating in between as well. Incredibly, I was still on one injection per day. I really wanted to prove I was a good worker and not have an employer consider my diabetes as a liability.

I started to learn the job, but was hindered by the clerk who was training me. She was limiting how much knowledge she was willing to share. In the meantime, I decided to take some night courses at the local college to increase my knowledge of Microsoft applications. I felt that I was being taken advantage of at my current job. It seemed as if the clerk training me felt threatened that I might want to take her job. She would handle the easy tasks and gave me the more difficult tasks or anything she didn't want to do.

My boss told me they were going to expand, and he was going to need an assistant to support their business accountant. I told him I was taking computer courses at night and that I understood the company would reimburse me for courses relevant to my job. He said they would cover three of the courses and he asked me if I would be interested in the new position. It would be supporting him and five field technicians doing travel arrangements, processing expense reports and updating spreadsheet schedules. I accepted the position and was hired as a permanent employee.

I worked closely with the accountant to learn the tasks and I was very good at my job. I grew my expertise in all of the applications and started to use them heavily in the office. One day I delivered a report to a manager who sat in the back office near the tool and die machines. As I left his office, my left foot slipped on some oil and I reached out and grabbed a hold of a metal bar on one of the machines. After catching myself, I thanked God I hadn't fallen or gotten seriously injured. When I got back to my desk, I noticed my left arm felt a bit stressed and stretched.

A few weeks went by and I started to have a little pain in my left shoulder. I ignored it, thinking it would go away. As I was approaching my one-year anniversary, I found out through the grapevine that upper management was planning to move the company to another location out of state. When I confirmed it was true, I immediately started looking for another position because I was not going to wait to be unemployed.

I sent my resume to several agencies and I landed a position in the Credit Marketing Department for a very large retailer with thousands of employees. I worked with three other assistants supporting different managers.

By this time, the pain in my left shoulder was constant. It continued getting worse and was gradually freezing up on me to the point that I could not move my shoulder easily.

I knew I had to do something. I needed to work to support myself and the diabetes. I realized I must have torn something in my left shoulder when I prevented that fall at my last job. It was too late to file a workman's comp claim and I never told anybody it happened to me. I had brushed it off because I didn't actually fall and never considered that I had injured myself. I continued to work at the new company, but because I was a temporary employee, I had to pay out of pocket for health insurance.

I made an appointment with an orthopedic doctor to check my shoulder, likely having to spend my entire salary to treat it. He took an x-ray and told me nothing was broken and told me to get an MRI which showed I had micro-adhesions in my left shoulder. I likely tore my shoulder then developed adhesions from it trying to heal. He also told me it was very common for diabetics to get frozen shoulders. I asked what he could do and he said I could try physical therapy but he couldn't guarantee I would get full range of motion. Naturally, I was upset with yet another hurdle to get over. I got a second opinion and after reading my results, this doctor immediately recommended surgery. When I asked about my chances for a complete recovery, he said there was no guarantee it would heal correctly due to the diabetes. I was even more upset. How would I be able to function? I was in constant pain and the slightest wrong move would trigger more pain. I took my reports and said I would think about it and left briskly. I decided to search the internet at work to look for solutions for frozen shoulders that didn't involve surgery. I came across a chiropractor's website that talked about their success in reversing frozen shoulders. He was Chinese and also practiced acupuncture. I decided to give him a call and make an appointment. When I called his office, I discovered they did not take my insurance so I needed to go on a payment plan. I didn't care, I needed my arm functional again and surgery was not an option. I decided to give him a chance.

I walked into his office and I had no idea what he would do. He explained he was going to manually break the adhesions with a chiropractic adjustment. He told me to sit upright on the chiropractic table and told me to take a deep breath in, then breathe out, and he did an adjustment to my shoulder. I heard and felt a pop in my shoulder and then felt an intense amount of pain. I screamed and felt like I saw stars – it was that painful. He asked if I was okay and I was silent for a minute. He said, "you will feel some relief instantly." He explained the process to me and we continued to talk for several minutes. The talking calmed me down. Then he told me to move my shoulder. For the first time in a year, I could slightly move my shoulder. It was amazing! This was progress.

I continued to see the chiropractor for over a year and also had several acupuncture treatments. I continued until my arm was more functional. It took many treatments and arm exercises on my own, but I was finally able to use my arm. I wasn't pain free but I saved myself from the agony of surgery and its consequences. I now had a better idea of how to treat things and not rely solely on modern medicine and could use alternative therapies when I needed them.

At work I occasionally had to deliver some reports to the other side of the building (approximately a half mile from one end to the other). There was a lot of glass windows and ceilings, and on sunny days, it was very bright. During one delivery, I started to notice that my vision in my left eye was slightly foggy. I worked closely with computers all day and thought maybe I needed an eye exam. My eye doctor did the typical exam and as he looked further, he told me I had a cataract but that it could be corrected with surgery. My heart began to pound. How could I have a cataract? Only old people get those. I was only 37 years old. Surgery? That was out of the question. I was not going to let anyone get near my eye with a scalpel. I thought, this is ridiculous! Everyone wants to fix me with surgery. I told the eye doctor I was going to wait. Again, I went to the internet to research alternative treatments for cataracts. After reading about some of the approaches, I came to the conclusion I was still functional. After all, I could see the eye chart, drive my car and see my computer at work. The only thing that bothered me was sunlight, so I just looked for the darkest sunglasses I could find. It was an easy and inexpensive solution.

Six months went by and I was not extended a full time offer, and I needed benefits, so I began looking again. I came across a computer software company that was looking for a regional administrator for their Midwest office that sounded great. The phone interview went very well, and the interviewer scheduled an in-person interview to meet with the hiring manager. The manager was impressed that I had skills with the IBM BPCS system. He asked me if I liked that system and, of course I said yes. He said he used that system himself, and he really liked it. At this point I had a pretty good feeling I was going to get the job. He asked if I had any more questions. I asked about the office hours and lunch hour. He said, "you want to go shopping at lunch? You can take two hours." I couldn't believe what I was hearing. He told me the job would require traveling a couple times a year to their bi-annual meetings. I felt hesitant about business travel and managing diabetes. After a second, I thought, why not? The interview ended and I graciously shook Hugh's hand. I told my mom I would need to travel at least twice a year and that the company offered health insurance benefits, including dental and vision. My mom said, "I don't think you should get a job where you have to travel." When I asked her why not she said, "what if something happens to you and you faint?" I said, "I will let them know I have diabetes." She said, "ok, well just think about it." Two days later I received the job offer. I was ecstatic as the salary was a thousand dollars more per year than what I asked for. After a month on the job, I would have great benefits and very good pay. I joined a health club so I could go swimming and move my shoulder even more which was helping very much. The diabetes was still there, but now I added some more exercise. I still had to watch the sugar intake and not overdo it.

I began working for the new company and I had my own office. As a software company they naturally had the most current software for everything, including Outlook, Excel, Word, PowerPoint, and MS Project as well as their own sales contract system. An administrator from the West Coast office came in to train me. Although she looked a little road weary, we set up to begin my training. Shortly after we started, I tried to move closer to the screen and accidentally hit the power button with my foot and shut down the computer. I said, "what happened?" Marcia laughed and said, "your foot hit the power button." I was glad she laughed and did not yell at me, it made me feel more at ease. Marcia said she liked me and we talked casually for a while. I brought up the fact that I had diabetes and I needed to eat lunch at a certain time. I wasn't going to hide my diabetes anymore. Marcia didn't seem to mind and it didn't affect the conversation at all.

After a month on the job, I received my health insurance benefits along with dental, vision and life. The company plan provided great coverage for my insulin and supplies. It was so nice that I didn't have to worry about health insurance coverage anymore.

The job was going well and it was by far the most enjoyable role I had ever experienced. I assisted in preparing presentations for the sales team, helped to put together contracts, learned the latest software applications and also participated in tradeshows with the sales team. The sales team would take me out to lunch at least once a week to restaurants near the office. The food was delicious, but it was very high carbohydrate, calorie laden food and my blood sugars would soar a few hours after eating. I loved the indulgence, but it was killing me. I couldn't resist the desserts either. If only I didn't have diabetes to worry about. I frequently had to give myself another injection once I got home.

As the months went by, and I increased my knowledge about the job and software products, Marcia asked me to participate in a software tradeshow in Chicago along with two other assistants. The first evening, after the tradeshow, I ordered a pasta dish in an Italian restaurant chosen by the Vice President. When the waiter brought it to me, it was piled so high I couldn't believe it. The Vice President said "enjoy and eat!!" I ate slowly to look like I was eating all evening. A few hours later I felt tired and nauseated. I was hoping to get back to the hotel soon to give myself an injection, but I didn't get to the room until after 10:30 p.m. and my blood sugar was 400 mg/dl. I was in ketoacidosis so, with a shaky hand I quickly gave myself about five extra units of insulin and prayed I wouldn't have low blood sugar that night. I heard a bunch of salesmen who were right next door and they were still drinking and playing cards. Needless to say, I didn't get much sleep. The next day I was on my feet for almost eight hours helping customers and by the end I had a terrible back ache, but it was a successful show. When I got home, I took time to recuperate and didn't eat much or do a whole lot.

The job was going well and I started to make better money so I bought my first laptop. The internet was available, so I began to research more about diabetes and looked for a cure. After being diagnosed with cataracts, I was hoping to find a cure before I would experience any more complications. I read a story about a middle-aged diabetic man who qualified for a pancreas transplant. His daughter wrote about how grateful she was that her father was cured of diabetes with the transplant and no longer required insulin shots or special diets. I decided to contact the company that was doing the transplants. The company responded and asked me to send my latest results for my blood and kidney function. My blood urea nitrogen (BUN) level was only 8 mg/dl which was too low for a pancreas transplant. They were only doing transplants on people with extreme or critical problems and my diabetes was not severe enough. They also emphasized that I would need to be on immunosuppressant drugs for the rest of my life to prevent rejection of the new pancreas. The drugs could suppress my immune system and I would be likely be more susceptible to infections or cancer. It was a disappointment as I hoped to have a chance to be free of diabetes.

I heard about a "Walk for Diabetes" event and my mom agreed to do the walk with me. I wanted to meet some people and see if there was something new to learn about diabetes. After the walk, I looked around at all the sponsors and booths when I saw Miss America 1999, who had diabetes. I got a chance to talk to her and told her I was a long-term diabetic – 35 years at the time. I told her it was great to meet someone who had shared the agony of diabetes. It was an honor to meet her and I hoped she would be a strong advocate for a diabetes cure.

My company was holding their annual sales meeting in New Orleans. Everyone could bring a guest so I brought my mom. We had never been to Louisiana before. I wondered how I was going to survive all the meals there, as I didn't know what I would be eating or when. I always had to have some quick sugar in my purse in case of hypoglycemia. I could easily disappear to the rest room and quickly drink something.

Once we arrived in New Orleans, I met up with two other sales assistants from the East and West Coast. The first day of the sales meeting, I kept looking at my watch to see how soon before I could eat lunch. I was a nervous wreck thinking about my diabetes. I excused myself so I could go check my blood sugar and it was still high from breakfast. I went back to my seat and grabbed a diet soda. Soon lunch was served which was a tray of salads and sandwiches. I tried to pick out something that wasn't too big. I didn't want to feel sick from eating. After the meeting all of us went back to the hotel to change for dinner. I took insulin with me, and we went to an old Louisiana home dating back to the 1800's that had been converted into a restaurant. The menu consisted of things like jambalaya and crawfish. I stuck with a regular meat and potato dish and had a little of the dessert. I hoped I wouldn't be flying high later with ketoacidosis. I also tucked a couple of rolls in my purse in case I needed something before going to bed.

I tried to get through the rest of the sales meeting without incident. Every evening we went to another restaurant that had rich foods that were not diabetes-friendly. I continued to eat small amounts to keep me out of the emergency room and I imagined how great it would be to enjoy eating those foods without thinking about it. I could have eaten like a king, but really couldn't enjoy a lot of good southern cooking. My mom and I decided to stay an extra day to see the sights before we went home. We took a ride on the Creole Queen on the Mississippi river, walked around in the New Orleans shops and visited an old plantation. After the trip I was exhausted from my poor diet and poor sleep. It was quite an experience traveling for work and with higher blood sugar, I ended up with another yeast infection. I had to be on an antifungal yet again for seven days.

The company decided to have all the employees trained on new software. This was a two-week program at their headquarters in California. I had to go and I couldn't get out of it. When I got home I asked my mom what I should do. How could I even survive there with diabetes?" My mom said "Tell them you will only go for a week. I will go with you, but I will stay out of sight and no one will see me."

I booked the flight for both myself and my mom and we flew to California. When we arrived at the hotel, it was quiet and I didn't see anyone I knew. Once I unpacked and settled in, I contacted Marcia and joined her at the training. I told my mom to make sure nobody saw her.

Each evening we went to restaurants including a popular seafood place in Malibu, frequented by movie stars. The meals were a little healthier with smaller portions, so it was easier to accommodate my diet. The next evening, we went to a five-star restaurant where the food was more decadent, so I was careful not to order too much. I was amazed to see a lot of older women there with face lifts and tight clothing. They had no idea how lucky they were to be in good health. All I could do is stare. I looked at my meal and hoped for the best with my blood sugar.

We also visited Hollywood, the Chinese Theatre, and took a ride up the coast to Malibu which was a nice sightseeing trip. The week went by fast and I was ready to go home. As we waited outside for the airport shuttle, Marcia spotted me from inside the hotel and started to come toward me. My mom noticed and said, "I better get on so she doesn't see me." I waited for Marcia and we quickly said our goodbyes. A salesman from the East Coast I'd met earlier in the week was going to the airport on the same shuttle. He helped me carry my suitcase and then sat down next to me. My mom sat across from us and tried not to stare. We were talking and he told me where he was from. When we arrived at the airport, he helped me again, then grabbed my mom's suitcase. He had noticed she had the same last name as mine. I got nervous but I laughed it off and said, "she probably has the same last name as mine - a coincidence." My mom said "Thank you" and we started walking separately to check in at the airport. The salesman then started looking suspiciously at both of us. I gave my mom a look so she wouldn't give me away and he wouldn't figure out we were together. The salesman wanted to see if he could get on the same flight as me on the way home and then catch a connection to the East Coast. There was no availability. Phew! I walked with him to his gate and talked a bit and then said I had to go. I finally found my gate, but it was final call and I was the last one to board the plane before it left. My mom was in a panic, but I made it and quickly took my seat next to her.

It was summer and I was looking forward to finally have some vacation time. My region did very well that quarter in software sales and I had helped one of the salesmen put together all the materials to secure a million-dollar contract. I learned a lot during the process and I was looking forward to working there for several more years. In the accounting department, things were looking much different. The company spent over a million dollars just on air travel for employees and now they were looking to make adjustments somewhere in the company. I didn't like the sound of it, but I assumed my job was secure. A few weeks later, Marcia called me on a Thursday and said I needed to book a mandatory flight to the East Coast for a meeting on Monday morning. I asked if she was going, and she told me no. I was suspicious about this last-minute trip. I then found out one of the lower performing salesmen in my region needed to go too. I started to get a feeling in the pit of my stomach, and it wasn't due to diabetes. I made reservations and decided to fly in on Saturday and stay at my uncle Oleg's house until Monday. Mom and I arrived and uncle Oleg picked us up.

He was happy to see us, but he didn't appreciate the short notice. We spent the weekend at his home with his wife and teenage girls. My uncle took us to the seashore to walk around. It was lunch time and I felt like my blood sugar was dropping. With all the rush, I forgot to put something in my purse and asked my mom if she had any juice. My uncle right away said to my mom, "Why are you carrying around juice for her? Isn't she old enough to do that? She's a big girl." My mom got angry and said, "you don't understand, if she faints it could be serious. Did you forget she has diabetes?" For a moment I was trying to enjoy myself and forget about diabetes. I knew I could count on my mom if I needed her. My uncle just shook his head and thought what my mom was doing was wrong. He just didn't understand. The average person just doesn't understand that things can go bad very quickly with diabetes. Luckily, mom did have some juice, so we continued to enjoy the day.

I woke up Monday morning and put on my suit for the meeting. I walked in and saw a few salesmen. I didn't have a smile on my face because I sensed there was bad news being delivered to us. The assistant from the East Coast was there. I remembered what a good time we had a few months back and now it felt like we were attending a funeral. There were about eight of us and one salesman from the East Coast said we were probably going to lose our jobs. It made sense. I was trying to get a grip on myself before hearing the news. A few minutes later, the Vice President arrived looking very professional but with a cold demeanor. He had several envelopes that were filled with thick paperwork. He explained that due to recent financial issues, the company was closing down the Midwest and East Coast region and that those of us present were all getting laid off. I felt a storm of emotions going through my body starting with the fact that I would lose my health insurance. The company would provide outplacement services for us as well as two months' severance pay. After the meeting we all said our goodbyes and how great it was to have worked together. I walked out of the building and waited for my uncle to pick me up. He asked me how the meeting went and I just said "okay". I didn't want to tell him I had lost my job. I was embarrassed. This was my first experience with a lay-off and I didn't know how to deal with it. I was feeling really down on the flight home.

The following week after we got home, I called the outplacement service. The manager helped me write my resume and put it together professionally. He told me he never imagined he would land the job he had. His parents were poor farmers that came to the United States and he was able to achieve his dream of doing 100% better than his parents. That gave me drive to do better as I looked for my next job. I would learn how to ask for more, and not to settle for less. I secured a job six weeks later with a large company that was nearly 100 years old. I got four thousand more dollars per year having learned how to negotiate in an interview. Now it was a matter of learning the new job and succeeding at it.

I was doing well in my new position, but the employees were not as friendly as the ones at my last job. I felt like a worker bee and that was it. I didn't tell anyone I had diabetes because I was concerned about discrimination. As my workload increased, it became increasingly more difficult for me to see the numbers on the white screen. My reading glasses didn't make a difference and my cataracts were getting worse. Several weeks later, I didn't think I could continue to do well at this job with my vision changing. I decided to look for another job that didn't require intense computer work. I was able to find another job working for another large company as an Executive Assistant for a Vice President. I was happy, but concerned about how my vision would be on this job. I updated my glasses and, luckily, I could perform my work. I got to know all the other Executive Assistants that worked on the floor, all of them friendly, with the exception of two older women that had worked there for many years. I frequently had to leave my desk and walk a few yards away to get answers to my various questions. The company president required every phone call be answered, and that nothing go to voicemail. I could barely be away from my desk, so there was hardly time to be a diabetic. I tried to keep my blood sugar higher, so I wouldn't risk fainting. My only refuge was diet soda, and I drank a lot of it. Supporting a vice president was demanding and I could make no mistakes. My boss missed an important meeting once, and I was to blame. I apologized, but it wasn't enough and I was terminated. I didn't see it coming and I was back to the job search.

Chapter Seven

Family Health Matters

My mom turned 59 and she was very busy with her job working at the school district. After having dinner, she often complained about her stomach hurting and feeling sick. Every evening, she fell asleep on the couch around 7:00 p.m., while I watched TV. I figured it was due to job stress. After seeing her doctor and undergoing some tests, it was evident that she too had diabetes. She had the option of taking medication or following a strict diet to manage her blood sugar. This news made me fearful and anxious. Would this shorten her life? Was this the beginning of her decline?

Right away, my mom went on a strict diet and lost at least 20 pounds. She was able to avoid taking medication for the rest of the year, and seemed to be doing very well. I was pleased that she was so compliant. She was not a diabetic in denial. She had lots of experience from my lifetime of diabetes and knew how serious this was.

At this point, my career was in turmoil. I had one mishap after another with my jobs and my vision was an issue. I was concerned about my mom's health and I didn't have insurance coverage for myself. I began to look again for jobs in the newspaper and also online. I came across an ad for a contracting job with a very large corporation. It was a step down from all my previous jobs, but I had to go for it. I passed all the computer tests and the contracting company had placed me in a one-month contract working for a Director in the Procurement Department.

On the first day, my boss came over to my cubicle after I had settled in and said "Hello, I'm Mr. Brady, the Director." I turned around and saw a well-dressed man with glasses. He said, "Welcome to the procurement department." I wasn't going to jeopardize my position by telling anyone I was a diabetic. I hid my blood glucose testing machine by taking it to the ladies' room or hiding it under my desk. I kept tabs on how my blood sugar was all day, so I wouldn't get the dreaded lows. My mom's diabetes was on my mind, and I called her a few times a day to check up on her.

Mr. Brady always complemented me on my work, and said I was sharp. A few weeks went by and some inevitable changes were occurring. The company had merged with another business and there were going to be job cuts. Mr. Brady told me they were offering him an exit package for his years of service at the company. I knew my contracting job would soon be over and I didn't have another one lined up after that. One of the hiring managers said she was going to be affected by the job cuts, but she was going to forward my resume to another Director that was looking for an assistant. The Director was interested in my resume and wanted to set up an interview which took place fairly quickly.

I came home feeling melancholy. Based on my previous experiences, I expected the worst and felt certain I wasn't going to get the job. My anxiety went through the roof and I paced back and forth in the house.

Remarkably, I received a call from Human Resources and they were offering me the position, if I was still interested. I answered in a calm voice, "yes, I would be interested." This was a small pay cut for me, but I knew the benefits would be excellent. When I hung up the phone, I felt like I won the lottery and ran up to my closet to get my wardrobe ready for the following week. I had to look absolutely professional. Several days later, I received a large gift basket wrapped in plastic with a bow and a tag that said "Welcome to the Company". I had to pinch myself to see if this was really happening. I felt nothing short of euphoric.

I started my new job the following week and my new boss, Mrs. Sharp, stopped over. I helped her move into her new office and once we settled in everything seemed to go well.

I was in charge of helping a team of 180 staff with all their administrative needs which was a lot of responsibility. I decided to skip getting an interim health insurance plan until I was eligible for benefits in 30 days, and prayed I wouldn't need medical attention during that time. Miraculously, the company paid 100% of my medical coverage. All my medications; insulin, thyroid medication, and blood glucose testing strips were covered –I did not need to pay a dime. This was a welcome relief.

Several months into the job, Mrs. Sharp was having a staff meeting out of state. It was about an hour flight and I was required to accompany her, take meeting notes and distribute them to the senior technical directors. I told my mom and she started to panic. I said I needed to go, but that I would return the same day. She told me to make sure to take snacks and take my insulin and syringes with me, just in case. I packed a purse that looked like a computer laptop case and put everything in there. This was the first time I traveled by myself on company business and I prayed that my medication and syringes went through security, and luckily, everything went smoothly.

We arrived at the company location and the meeting went as planned. My blood sugar was elevated just from the stress and I felt tired so I drank a lot of diet soda. After the meeting was over, Mrs. Sharp wanted to speak to me in private in a nearby office. One hundred thoughts went through my head, what did I do wrong? I sat down in a chair across the desk from her while she proceeded to compliment me on my work and tell me I was getting a $2000 per year raise. I couldn't believe it. I thanked her graciously and she said, "enjoy!"

My mom was overjoyed when I told her, and we were both happy that the future looked brighter and that things seemed to be going so well.

I was 39 years old with 36 years of diabetes under my belt. I learned of a Diabetes Expo that was being held downtown and thought that my mom and I might attend and learn something new, including information about potential cures. After a quick pass by all of the exhibitors, there didn't seem to be anything new or groundbreaking. However, I came upon a booth that had information about islet transplants that were already being done to cure diabetes. This type of transplant involves placing healthy cells from a donated pancreas into a diabetic's pancreas in order to restore normal function, enabling the body to make insulin. I asked about immunosuppressant drugs and the people staffing the booth verified that anti-rejection medications continue to be an important part of treatment following any transplant. I learned that the weight restrictions were less stringent and I decided to take some information. My insurance would cover transplants, but I was still concerned about the drugs I would need to take for the rest of my life.

I began to be very busy with my job and assuming more responsibility. There was an endless amount of things to learn about technology in my department. I started drinking more diet soda and I would sneak in some sweets almost every afternoon after lunch. It was a small reward, and I knew I was killing myself in the process. Like most offices, sweets were always available - donuts, birthday cake and more. I had to draw on my willpower, and it didn't always work as my blood sugar often ran over 200 mg/dl. One injection was not enough so I had to bring fast acting insulin and syringes to work and make sure no one saw me inject myself. Sometimes I would sneak into a conference room and give myself an injection, if needed, then walk out nonchalantly. The company installed instant messaging on our computers and I was the contact for all the members of the team. My stress levels were increasing and at the end of the day I was exhausted.

One day at work I received an email about a fundraising walk for diabetes research. The walk was held in downtown Chicago and my mom and I each tapped into our co-workers for sponsorship. The event was held on a beautiful warm September day. Hundreds of people participated which reminded me how this disease had impacted so many lives. Participating in this event made me feel much less alone. I collected some brochures from exhibitors at the walk and one of them happened to be about insulin pumps. When I first read about them years ago, they were very expensive and the size of a brick. These new pumps were much smaller, and could be worn easily on a belt or waistband. I decided to give them a call, thinking I might qualify. What a relief to know I may not have to inject myself every day!

On Monday, I contacted my health insurance company, and they told me that they would cover the insulin pump 100%. All I needed was an order from my doctor. I was stunned! Retail cost for the pump was about $6,000.00, but I was fortunate to have full coverage of the expense. I began to imagine life without needles and it was exciting. The pump did require changing after a few days, but that was minor in comparison to poking myself with a needle every day. It would be relatively easy to hide under my clothing, too. In just a week I received the insulin pump and management of my diabetes was notably easier and certainly less painful.

The next day was Tuesday, September 11, 2001. I had no idea what was about to occur and when I arrived at my desk and flipped the page on my desk calendar, I literally said under my breath, "What is going to happen today?" I was thinking about my responsibilities, and what would need my immediate attention. I had just settled in at my desk, and the budget analyst called me from St. Louis and said, "the World Trade Center just got attacked - an airplane hit one of the towers." He had prior military training and said, "This is an act of war!" I was a bit confused and said, "could it be just a big accident?" He replied, "This is no accident!!"

My boss arrived shortly thereafter and she had also heard on the radio that one of the twin towers in New York was attacked. I was in a huge building with 4,000 employees at the time and apprehension set in. I pulled up the story online and sure enough there was a picture with a plume of black smoke surrounding one of the towers. I printed a copy and showed my boss. She had a blank look on her face. One of the assistants in the department came over to my desk and started telling me what happened and how the second tower had also been hit. It was a horrible scene and now I felt panic. What if our building is next? Like everyone in the country, we soon learned the pentagon was hit with major damage and a fourth plane had been hijacked and went down in a field. My co-worker was in shock and said, "I can't stay here, I'm going home." I wanted to leave as well, but my boss didn't say anything, and I had too much to lose if I got fired for leaving, so I stayed. The company made an announcement over the intercom about the situation and a television was set it up in the employee mezzanine so everyone could see what was happening. I tried to take some breaks to watch, but I had to focus on my work. Soon I realized I was safe at work and stayed until 5:00 p.m. When I arrived at home, both my mom and I watched the day's horror unfold on all the news channels. I began to cry seeing that my beloved country had been attacked and things would never be the same. In the following weeks, there were various fundraisers held at work to raise money for needed supplies for the firefighters on site in New York.

With the arrival of my insulin pump and the supplies, I had something positive to focus on amidst all the chaos in the world. I was a little overwhelmed, however, a nurse would be coming over to set up the insulin pump and instruct me how to attach it. The nurse said I would still have low blood sugar and would need to monitor it very carefully. The insulin pump showed the amount of insulin I had remaining in my body, so I could adjust it based on my blood sugar reading. If my sugar was going lower, I could have some food or juice to compensate for it.

The first full day I was on the insulin pump, I checked my blood sugar two hours after I had eaten a meal. To my amazement, my blood sugar was 72 mg/dl. I believe this was the first time in my life I had a favorable reading after eating. I was really excited that I could now check how many units were remaining on the pump, and I could eat a little more if I wanted to. I could even have ice cream and pizza, once I learned how to compensate for it. This was nearly impossible on single manual injections and this meant a little more freedom from diabetes! I really loved how the pump changed my life. I made sure to take excellent care of this valuable asset for managing my diabetes.

The next Christmas, I allowed myself to have cookies, cakes, and pies and truly celebrate like everyone else. I went a little crazy at first and ate a lot of things that would have been forbidden previously. I indulged in regular soda once in a while, ice cream, potato chips, chocolate bars, and even milk shakes! It was okay for a while, but then my weight started to creep up as a result of my "treats".

After several months I felt so much better because I was more effectively managing my blood sugar levels. I had my first glyco-hemoglobin (A1C) test since starting the pump and my result was 6.5. Normal ranges for a non-diabetic were 5.5 and I was very close. It was quite a change from years past where at one point my A1C was 11.0. Learning to control myself with food was hard while allowing myself access to all the foods that were forbidden in the past. Gaining weight was not a good idea either and I had gained 10 pounds since being on the insulin pump.

I was very fortunate to have good medical insurance. I had access to specialists and could also get supplemental insurance to cover any critical needs, like transplants. An islet transplant was always in the back of my mind and the fact that it might be an option for me. I was reminded how invaluable my job and its medical benefits were to me and how taking care of my diabetes depended on it.

In 2002, my mom decided she wanted to sell the house and move into a better neighborhood. I started looking online for homes and visiting some available properties. My mom fell in love with a newer house in a quieter neighborhood. As I considered my mom's life and how hard she worked and all of the struggle she experienced, I felt she deserved something nice. The next month, we were approved and moved in to our new home. She loved working in the yard and planting flowers. Things seemed to be getting better for both of us.

Several months after our move, I noticed my vision got even worse. I had to keep changing my prescription for thicker and thicker lenses. My eye doctor said my cataracts were worse, but they weren't "ripe enough" yet to do the surgery. I wanted to hold off with surgery until absolutely necessary and I kept praying that miraculously my vision would improve on its own. I began searching online for holistic cures. I decided to bring a magnifying glass to work and use it inconspicuously when nobody was looking or passing by my desk. This could help me get by and I certainly didn't want to tell anyone at work what was happening to my vision. Everyone thought I was fine, and my thick glasses were simply for deteriorating vision due to old age.

My mom always knew what was going on with me and was my constant support. She also had a slight case of cataracts, but could still function well. I began to fear losing my sight which would have devastated me. I was only 41 and thought I would fall apart if that happened. I couldn't help but think that with the use of the insulin pump and tighter blood sugar control, I could halt the cataracts. Driving home after work, I had a hard time seeing the street signs. I tried not to drive at night which was getting to be almost impossible. The headlights from oncoming traffic looked like sparks and blurred my vision until they passed by. I could still function during the day, but it was getting increasingly difficult. Once cataracts become debilitating, surgery is the only answer.

My mom's diabetes was getting worse. After four years of managing Type 2 through diet only, she was finally at a point where she needed to go on insulin. She began to have blood sugar into the 200's, and insulin was the only answer. She already had years of knowledge about diabetes from raising me and I believed she would be careful to manage her condition. She stayed very active, walked during her lunch hour, and did yard work and cleaning around the house. I was concerned about her, and now that she was going on insulin, there was always a possibility of low blood sugar.

Despite the doctors' opinion, I continued to search out answers for cataracts that didn't include surgery. I found a website selling natural supplements for cataracts that made the astonishing claim that they would "Get rid of those clouds in your eyes". It was worth a try. I purchased the supplements and took them for several months but did not see any difference.

My boss often sent me last minute projects to do with tight deadlines that had me scrambling to finish on time. I put an Excel spreadsheet together with numbers that I thought were correct. My boss sent it back to me and said "this isn't right, please fix it". I had no idea what she was talking about. I looked it over several times and then asked her what the problem was. It turned out that some of the numbers were yellow on a white background, and I could not see them on the spreadsheet due to my poor vision. She had to point it out to me. I felt like a fool, but I honestly couldn't see it and I couldn't tell her why. I deeply apologized and said I would take care of it. I took my magnifying glass and made sure everything balanced and looked perfect. This event really hit me hard and I was under more stress now due to my vision.

Summer was approaching and my mom wanted to plan a vacation to have some fun. Why not? I needed a break and there was a Ukrainian Festival going on in Toronto, Canada. My mom wanted to go so I made the plane reservations.

When we arrived, we did some sightseeing and it felt like I was looking at most things through a fog. At the festival, there were displays set up that I had to get very close to in order to see. I could see the ocean and larger things like buildings and furniture, but faces in the crowd were not discernable. We went to a stage show in the evening and my mom was enjoying the dancers and singers, but I basically stared into space. My vision made it impossible to enjoy.

After the festival was over, my mom wanted to drive to the Canadian side of Niagara Falls to show me where she and my father spent their honeymoon in 1959. We arrived at the falls and I was taken aback by the enormity of water coming down over the cliff and the powerful sound. I couldn't see it clearly, but I wanted to enjoy it so much. My mom said, "look there's a rainbow in the falls!" I said, "I see it, but I wish I could have seen the whole beauty of it." In my mind I thought this was probably the last vacation I would go on before I couldn't see anymore.

When I got home, I looked for a specialist that was covered under my medical insurance. I found a professor at the University Medical School who specialized in cataracts who was also a surgeon. I wanted to choose someone who knew what they were doing.

I met the eye doctor, but I couldn't see her face very well. She looked scary to me. My mom said she was pretty and all I saw was a distorted face. She took my health history and seemed amazed that I had diabetes since 1964. She dilated both my eyes and checked for glaucoma, but the pressure in my eyes was normal. Following the exam she said "you have a classic case of sugar induced cataracts, a direct result of diabetes". She said I would first need to see a retinal specialist and then she could perform surgery to fix the cataracts. I asked her how bad they were and she said, "We could wait, but it is up to you". I left the appointment knowing that if I didn't do the surgery, I surely would go blind. Because of having diabetes and all of the associated challenges, I was sure it would not go well.

After seeing the retinal specialist, my test results were favorable and my retina looked fantastic. He said "this scan of your retina looks like you have a retina of a 12-year old!!" I simply couldn't believe it. He gave the go ahead to have the cataract surgery.

At work I continued having a hard time seeing people's faces from a distance. Co-workers going to lunch in the cafeteria recognized me and waived. I smiled trying to figure out who they were and pretended I knew.

On the way home from work that week, traffic was stopped due to a car accident and a police officer was directing traffic off my route. I panicked and called my mom on my cell phone. I said, "I don't know what street I just turned on and where it goes. I can't see the sign and I don't know how to get home!" My mom was also in a panic. I couldn't tell her where I was or where I was going. It was almost sunset and I was crying. She said, "Don't worry, just look around, maybe you'll recognize something on the road." "There are nothing but trees on both sides of the road", I said in a crying voice. As I approached the next intersection, I heard an ambulance going towards the hospital so I turned on the same street. I was able to figure out where I was and I found the way home. I came into the house and my mom hugged me. She had been extremely worried.

Despite this frightening episode I continued to struggle at work and mistakes were not hard to make. I was on the verge of blindness yet I was still in denial about the surgery and the thought of having my eyes cut made me cringe. I thought back to dissecting a cow's eye in high school biology class. Enough said.

In the summer of 2006, I was already contemplating a pure white seeing eye dog that would lead me around. There goes my job and starting to be a constant burden to my mom. I scheduled another appointment with the eye surgeon. Dr. Kay was very nice and when she examined me, she said "dear, I think it's time for you to get the surgery. Did you want me to schedule it?" I asked about the complications from the surgery and she said there was a 1% chance that there might be problem and she felt the surgery would go well. I bit the bullet and nodded my head yes and said, "Let's schedule the surgery."

I was feeling depressed and all I kept thinking about was the surgery, and how it would go wrong, and my future seeing eye dog. The nurse came in and explained the procedure for the surgery and scheduled a date. On the ride home, I thought about how I was going to explain this to my boss since I would need to be off of work for one week.

I came into work and called my insurance company for pre-authorization for surgery. About an hour after I talked to them, my boss sent me an instant message that she wanted to see me in her office. I felt my heart drop.

I knocked on her door and sat in front of her desk. She said "What's going on with you? The insurance company called me to verify surgery?" I let out a big sigh. I said, "I've been putting this off for a while, but I'm going to need cataract surgery." "Cataract surgery?", she said, "Aren't you too young for that?" I said, "Well, cataracts run in my family. My two uncles had the surgery and my grandmother had cataracts as well." "What causes it?" she said. "I have no idea", I said, "All I know is that it runs in my family". There was no way I was going to tell her my diabetes caused it. She said, "Well okay, I'm sorry to hear about it. Look for an assistant to fill in for you while you are out" she said. "No problem", I said. I went back to my desk and was relieved she believed my cataract story. I had to wait three more weeks until the surgery and even though I wasn't looking forward to the operation, it was incredibly difficult to function. I only had 20% visual acuity.

It was the day before surgery, and I looked at my mom's face to try and remember her features. My mom was just as apprehensive as I was. I was her only child, and she knew how much I had already been through. Only she would understand. In the morning my uncle Paul came by to pick us up and take us to the hospital. The nurse gave me a gown to change into and took my vital signs. I wore my insulin pump into surgery and my blood sugar was 160 mg/dl. After I got on the table, the nurses tied my arms down and strapped my head down with tape. They covered my eye with Betadine solution, and a topical anesthetic to prevent my eye from moving during surgery and then draped my face with a round opening for the eye. I needed to be awake during the surgery. All I could think of was not being able to escape in case of an emergency! The nurses turned on some loud rock music in the operating room and my blood pressure started going up. Dr. Kay noticed my vital signs and with a firm voice told them to shut off the music. I was relieved. Once they started to do the procedure, I saw a hazy, pink and turquoise light over my eye. I couldn't see anything else. I didn't know when they made the cut and extracted the old lens. I didn't say a word and I felt nothing. At one point, Dr. Kay asked me "Honey are you okay?" I said in a short quick voice "yes". She said "It will be over real soon".

I was only in surgery for about an hour, but it felt like an eternity. I wondered what my blood sugar was, since my stomach was empty. When they completed the surgery, they put a bandage on the eye and wheeled me into a recovery room. I felt a little dizzy, but relieved. After I was wheeled in, the nurse carefully took off my bandage. To my astonishment, I could see clearly. I could see the beautiful nurse's face in detail. I saw the red and white tiles on the wall. The colors were bright and clear as day. I made it through and it was successful!

The nurse was concerned about my blood pressure. She said it was very high in surgery which made sense as I was extremely nervous. The nurse said, "Your mom wants to see you, she's very concerned." My mom came into the room and said, "are you alright?" She saw me looking at her without any bandages. I said, "Mom, I see your face!!" I was never so grateful in all my life as I was to Dr. Kay. In a little while, I was taken out of recovery and my mom helped me put on my clothes. I was so excited about the results, I could not contain myself. I absorbed the environment through my new eye. It was a miracle! I was smiling and joking with the nurses. Dr. Kay came to see me and I thanked her, but she abruptly said "See you tomorrow for post op!" and ran to the next procedure. I had sutures in my eye and it felt itchy, like I had an eyelash in there. I was told the sutures would eventually bind and heal and the nurse gave me dark glasses to wear for 24 hours.

I got in the car and couldn't believe how well I could see. My vision was 20/20 in my left eye again. I was excited to see the street signs, perfectly clearly again. Every road we passed, I yelled out the name. When I arrived home, I looked at the house, the furniture, the pictures on the wall, the plants and the yard through the window. The garage door was open and I could see a female jogger go by in a bright hot pink top. Everything was so new to me, and I was giddy.

I looked more closely at my mom's face and noticed that she had aged. I hadn't been able to see well for almost nine years, and it was hard to see how her face got older.

The next day, my uncle Paul drove both my mom and I to the hospital for a post op appointment and my vision was better than 20/20. Dr. Kay said my eye looked very good and I could return to work. As I drove to the office the neighborhood looked so lovely to me, although the traffic was not. No one but my boss knew I had the surgery. When I arrived at my cubicle, I almost didn't recognize it. My desk was full of huge dust bunnies. I had been sitting at that desk for hours on end, not knowing how dirty it was. I was embarrassed.

My boss arrived at work. She said "Hi! How are you?" in a high-pitched enthusiastic voice. I said, "Really great, the surgery went well." I saw her unfuzzy face for the first time and she looked older than I thought. She said, "You were missed around here", and sure enough my inbox had several hundred emails to catch up on.

At lunchtime I walked over to the cafeteria and really enjoyed looking around. I recognized some people and waived to them. I reminded myself that it was more important than ever to stay on a diet to keep my blood sugar in line. I wanted my incision to heal correctly. The other eye still had a cataract and I would need surgery eventually. Being able to see made shopping a joy. Once I was able to see I noticed clothes in my closet weren't as nice as I thought they were.

I went to a local apple festival with my aunt and two younger cousins. It was crowded and I found myself amazed to see all the faces as I looked around. My young cousin, Andrew who was eight years old at the time, asked me if I could see better, and if the surgery hurt. I said, "yes, I could see better, and, no, it didn't hurt one bit." I gave him a little hug for caring so much. My cousins got some ice cream pops and I just watched them enjoy it.

It was a new world for me, and I was able to enjoy taking pictures again. At Christmastime, I snapped away with my camera and took many photos of my relatives. Everyone seemed to be older and my little cousins looked cuter than I'd remembered. I had a sense of renewal with my repaired eye and was grateful to God that I could see.

At 66 my mom was still working and I was hoping she would start to get ready for retirement. She kept telling me, there's still a mortgage to pay.

As summer approached, my mom started wearing her flip flops as they were the most comfortable for her feet. I suddenly noticed a mass on her left ankle and when I mentioned it, she said she was starting to have pain there. Foot care for diabetics is critical so I said, "Don't you ignore that!" I made an appointment for her with an orthopedic doctor I used to work for who said it needed to be removed. He had a twin brother who was a surgeon that specialized in tumors. When we saw the specialist, he could not determine what the mass was, and didn't know if it was cancer. The pain was getting worse, and surgery was scheduled. I was likely more frightened than my mom was. As my mom was wheeled into surgery, I gave her a kiss on the cheek and then sat in the waiting room where I prayed almost the entire time. I brought a book, but I watched TV instead in the waiting room. I kept an eye on my blood sugar and brought snacks, just in case I was going low. Finally, after 2 ½ hours, a nurse came by to tell me she was out of surgery and doing fine. They told me there was a slight complication in that a nerve in her foot was tangled around the mass. I was concerned whether she would be able to use her foot or have difficulty walking.

My mom was awake and was trying to emerge from anesthesia. She was hooked up to machines and an IV drip of morphine. In the room, I slept next to her in an uncomfortable roll-away chair. I was too high strung to sleep and kept thinking about what would happen with the nerve in her foot. I kept looking at the clock on the wall and couldn't wait until morning.

The next day a physical therapist came into the room to train her to use a walker and kept forcing her to stand up and put weight on her foot. She was screaming, but the therapist kept pushing her and I was in agony watching this. This was so soon after the surgery. On the third day, my mom was released, and I had to drive her home. Somehow, I had to get her in the house. I parked outside by the garage and helped her hang on until we got in the door. I don't know how I made it through the whole ordeal, but I was glad she was home safe. After a week, my uncle took her to her follow up appointment. The whole foot was blue, and the doctor said it would take a while for the sutures to heal. He apologized for having to cut the nerve, but he could not remove the mass without doing that. The surgeon explained the test results and said it was not cancer, yet they could not determine the cause. I was relieved it was not serious.

After a few weeks, my mom got better and could return to work. I was concerned that with her diabetes, things could take a turn for the worse. A month went by and she started to develop dark nodules near the surgery site and had pain in her foot. She had another appointment to follow up with her surgeon and she insisted she could drive herself downtown. I felt uneasy about it, but she insisted she could do it, and I didn't need to miss any time at work. The whole day I was a nervous wreck. In the afternoon, my mom called me on her cell phone and said she got lost going home on the highway. I was in a panic. I wasn't that familiar with the downtown area, so I couldn't help her. She said, "It's okay, I'll exit and ask someone." Visions of disaster started going through my head. What if she ends up in a bad area? I felt guilty letting her go by herself and bad scenarios ran through my head. "Oh Lord", I said, "Please get her home." About 45 minutes later she called me and said, "I'm home." She said she stopped by a gas station and the attendant steered her to the right road. "Thank you God", I said.

The surgeon did not know why she was getting dark nodules that were breaking open on her ankle and referred her to an infectious disease specialist. I remembered my experience with the patient that came in to the office with gangrene. I told my mom to make an appointment right away, don't mess around with diabetes! The infectious disease specialist said, "we will get to the bottom of this" and put her on several rounds of antibiotics. The incision was starting to heal, but the nodules were still there. It was a big mystery. My mom still continued to work despite my encouraging her to retire. She absolutely had no intention of retiring and said, "I have to get my pension, I need to work." I just sighed.

About six months went by and mom was still getting the nodules. They would heal more quickly now, but the foot still looked rather purple. I kept my eye on it and was troubled that the infectious disease doctor had no answer about the cause. When spring came, I watched her work in the back yard and I could still clearly see the purplish ankle through the window. I felt like she was losing her mind and putting herself in harm's way. I suggested she wear a shoe instead of a sandal and she insisted the sandal was more comfortable. She loved being outside and I couldn't control her. Even though I had an enormous amount of experience with diabetes, I felt useless. If gardening was her little piece of joy, I wasn't going to stand in the way. Eventually she started mowing the lawn. There was no stopping her. A relative shared how their grandmother saved her foot from gangrene by rubbing Aloe Vera gel on it. My mom tried it and there was some improvement. The nodules on her foot would continue to come and go for about a year.

At the start of 2009 I started to notice the cataract in my right eye was getting worse and I knew I would need surgery but still wanted to wait awhile. The doctor said I needed to make a decision when it was really non-functional. I guess I was one of the lucky diabetics if that was my only complication and I knew what to expect.

It was getting more difficult to work for my boss and she was more demanding than ever. I attributed it to my taking a lot of time off from work and the medical problems my mom and I had. I could look for another job within the company, but that would take time I didn't have. I had wonderful benefits and I had hoped to retire from this company.

In the spring my mom did the usual gardening clean-up outside, removing debris from the winter, raking leaves and trimming bushes. One day when she was sitting on the couch, she raised her left arm and I saw a round, red circle with a dark spot in the middle of it. I said, "Did you get bit by something?" It looked like some sort of bug bite. She said, "Maybe when I was trimming bushes?" I said, "You didn't feel like you were being bitten by something?" She said, "No." Because it appeared to be a rather large bite, I told her to see her doctor immediately. It was a Saturday, and luckily the doctor would be able to see her in her office. There was no fooling around, especially with diabetes.

The doctor checked it and said it looked like a puncture wound. I said, "Really? It's not a spider bite or something, maybe a tick bite?" "No" she said. "I'll prescribe an antibiotic cream and let me know if it doesn't help." I said, "My aunt had a tick bite and her doctor prescribed antibiotics right away." My mom's doctor said, "There is no Lyme Disease in this area." I figured she was right since my aunt Nadia lived on the East Coast. We picked up the topical antibiotic cream and my mom used it as directed. In about a week the wound was gone.

I felt like I was overwhelmed with medical problems. I constantly worried about my mom and her health, and the fact that she was still working. My work required constant vigilance to keep up with all the software changes and years of preparing for strike duty should the union employees declare one. This would require the employees at the corporate offices to fill in for their roles. During those times, we were walking on eggshells. I was able to get a doctor's note saying that I had a condition that would not allow me to work in the field.

In October or 2009, my mom started to complain about cramps in her lower legs mostly when she fell asleep on the couch while watching TV. I told her she needed to increase her magnesium supplements. It didn't really help. Then she started to complain about headaches on the top of her head and back pain. I told her she was pushing herself and maybe she should retire already. I said, "You have diabetes, don't you understand? You need to take care of yourself!"

The winter was snowy and cold and I always worried about my mom driving to work, and I prayed she would be alright as her route included some curvy roads. It was Ground Hog's day in February and I watched her drive off to work in one-inch of snow. It was just slick enough to be a problem. I kept thinking how crazy she was to still keep working having turned 70 years old.

There was no use in trying to get her to retire, or even go on vacation for that matter. Later that day I saw a call come in that was my mom's cell phone. I immediately picked up the phone and in a somber pained voice I heard, "Lucy, I broke my wrist." I said, "What happened?" She said, "I have one of my co-workers here and he is going to take me to the emergency room." Her co-worker said she fell by her car. I asked him, "Was it slippery there?" I immediately thought of her ankle, and wondered if it gave out. I told him I would be there in about ½ an hour. I was frantic. I just knew something would happen. She was aging, had diabetes, and a weak foot. When I arrived at the emergency room, I said, "Mom, are you okay?" She said, "I was two steps away from my car door and I fell backwards". The emergency room doctor came in and said that the x-ray showed a fracture. He said they would wrap it, but we needed to follow up with an orthopedic doctor for a cast. My mom said her back was hurting and she needed to get off the table. When she stepped down, she said "I can't move my legs, my back is in so much pain, and my neck too." That night was awful. The doctor gave my mom medication to get her through the night, however I don't think either of us slept. The stress was rising.

On the third day, we arrived at the orthopedic practice. The doctor said her wrist was a clean break and it should heal fine without a problem. He applied a cast and said, "No work for several weeks". My mom made sure I knew she was going back to work when this healed. I thought she was crazy.

After a week, my mom was back to cooking with her other hand. I was constantly worrying about her and would call home several times a day to check up on her. She could not drive, so she was stuck in the house with the television. Because my mom wasn't going to let a broken wrist stop her, she decided to take out the garbage without my knowledge. One day I called her in the afternoon and she had fallen in the garage on top of her car license plate that was sticking out. She hurt her back and I was again taking time off to take her to the orthopedic doctor. The x-ray showed a non-displaced fracture on her back rib. She was given pain medication and was in so much agony for a few weeks. I still needed to keep my job and I could not stay home to take care of her. My stress level was exploding! I was facing another cataract surgery, was definitely taking too much time off from work, and my mom was in tough shape.

A few weeks went by and it was time to take off her cast. My mom did not go back to work and her manager at work tried to convince her to retire. She had used up all her accumulated vacation pay to make up for the time off. She retained a lawyer because she fell on her employer's property which had also caused her very painful back problems. My Godfather, Jaroslav would take her to a back-care specialty practice when she needed to go. I was grateful I got some help with caregiving, but this was only the beginning. My mom fell several more times and, as a result, she returned to using a walker to get around.

In July, I saw my ophthalmologist, Dr. Kay who determined my cataract was "ripe enough" to remove. I was very prepared for this surgery and I trusted Dr. Kay. The surgery seemed to go quickly and when we drove home, I noticed that my eye was not as clear as with the first surgery. The eye surgeon told me that she had to leave 10% of the cataract behind, to prevent eye damage. Within a few weeks, my focus got better, but it wasn't as good as the first eye. I could live with it because it was still much better that what I had before.

I hoped and prayed that my mom would recover from her back issues. She was okay for a few months, but then in October of 2010 she fell again and lost her memory for a few minutes. I was extremely scared and I took her to the emergency room. The doctor admitted her for a few tests which revealed some issues with her spine. They brought in an orthopedic back specialist to look at her case. They scheduled her for an epidural injection and I took her home the following day. It helped the pain for a while, but that was short-lived. Surgery would not be an option, especially with her diabetes. After another serious fall, she ended up being admitted to the hospital again. This time the doctor brought in a neurologist to check her, including the grip in her hands. He recommended an EMG test to check her nerve conduction. Her legs were getting stiff and hard, and she was in an incredible amount of pain. At the neurologist, my mom could barely get up on the exam table she was so stiff. He told us she had a lot of firing in her nerves and it was not a good sign. He asked how long she had been a diabetic. I said, about 11 years. He said, "She has a condition called Stiff-Man Syndrome (SPS). This happens with diabetes." There was a treatment for the condition and he said "this is one in a million." I gasped. He said "the protocol for this is called IVIG which includes intravenous drugs to trick the immune system not to attack itself." SPS is an autoimmune condition and her treatment started the following week. She was given a tranquilizer four times per day and an IVIG treatment once a week. Initially, there was no improvement.

In about two months, she started to walk very, very, slowly with the walker. I had some hope, but progress was slow. After every IVIG treatment she was wiped out and needed to lay down the rest of the day. One side of her face was very red and swollen. After six months of treatment and more research into SPS, I told her that Mayo Clinic had discovered the first case back in the 1950's. I made arrangements to go there. At Mayo, she had nearly every neurological test done as well as blood tests and scans. The antibody test was positive again for SPS, however, I thought maybe they had a cure. The Mayo neurologists recommended more drugs to suppress her immune system. They had many bad side effects, and my mom was already very fragile. The neurologists told her to continue with the IVIG treatment and take the additional immunosuppressant drugs. I didn't sleep well for months thinking about this situation. I had no time to think about my own diabetes or focus on my health. When we arrived home, I did some research into the immunosuppressants. I told my mom not to take the additional medications but she continued on with the IVIG. Her neurologist also prescribed physical therapy. She was also suffering with anxiety and it was worse than ever. She continued to fall and each time I felt like I was closer to a nervous breakdown. Every fall was a set-back and I wondered if she needed a wheelchair. My entire focus was on getting her well. It was affecting me and my job performance because I had to take a lot of time off to take her to appointments. She couldn't drive and I was overwhelmed taking care of everything.

I wondered what caused this - it just came out of nowhere. I refused to believe it was only tied to diabetes. Was age a factor? My mom had deteriorated so quickly, what was the trigger?

Chapter Eight

———— ∼∼ ————

How Can We Heal?

MY LIFE TOOK a big dive and I never felt happy after this. I couldn't focus on anything except my mom's welfare. I was depressed every day at work, and I couldn't really think straight anymore. I would come home and see her in pain, sometimes crying. I felt helpless and overwhelmed. My immune system started to get worse from all the stress. I started to get intestinal infections and my gut was a mess. I was in agony at work all the time. I ended up in the emergency room due to severe dehydration and ended up in intensive care for three days. My blood sugar was 450 mg/dl. My sodium levels were so low I needed to be on IV fluids and I was so sick, I was scared I wouldn't make it. My uncle brought my mom to stay at the hospital with me, but she needed care herself. My boss called me at the hospital to ask me how I was, but I couldn't tell her I was in intensive care due to diabetic ketoacidosis and severe dehydration. I told her I had food poisoning. After my electrolytes and blood sugar were stabilized, I was released to go home. I was drained for several weeks after that. When I returned to work, I always remembered to drink plenty of fluids.

After having SPS for two years, my mom decided to prepare her final Will. It was so painful to think about this. She put together her last wishes and we saw a lawyer to draw up the paperwork. The thought of losing her to a horrible disease was unthinkable to me. I didn't know how to live with the thought, but I had to come to terms with it.

We did everything we were told to treat this disease. All the research said the same thing, autoimmune diseases can only be *managed*, there is no cure. The future for my mom, as well as myself, only looked bleaker. It was the lowest point in my life.

My mom continued with the IVIG therapy, tranquilizers, and physical therapy. It was status quo, no real change. One day just ran into the next and I didn't know how much longer she could survive. Later in the year she started to fall more and more, always falling backwards and injuring herself. I hired a caregiver to be with her during the day while I was at work which ate up half of my paycheck. I was happy she could talk to someone as she couldn't leave the house to socialize. I think it made her feel a bit happier to talk to someone.

In November, my uncle Paul drove my mom and I back to Mayo clinic for another evaluation. It turned out to be the same, no real help, no real answers. At this point I was fed up with the medical establishment. The neurologists there told her to take the immunosuppressant drugs as well as another drug to prevent bone loss. When I came home, I did more research. The drug side effects were worse than the drug's benefit. I told my mom not to take them yet. Mom had an eye doctor appointment the week after we arrived home from Mayo clinic. Her vision was getting worse. After the ophthalmologist checked her vision, she told us she was getting cataracts and would need surgery now. I was worried about her ability to handle surgery with this disease. We went home and talked about the situation and I scheduled an appointment with my own ophthalmologist for a second opinion about her vision. Since I had success with my eye doctor, she decided to use her for the surgery. When Dr. Kay checked her, she told her she had steroid induced cataracts, which had been used in combination with the IVIG treatment. I was more upset than ever. The drugs were doing more harm than good. I prayed she would have successful cataract surgery. At this point she could barely move and barely see.

If the surgery was not successful, I could not take care of her anymore. It was killing me inside. I continued to go to work and try to handle all the other problems at the same time. It was a very difficult and emotional time for me. Many times, I drove home from work and cried in my car which was the only time I could be vulnerable. My boss was always asking me how my mom was. I never had a good answer for her like – Oh! She's much better! It was always – she's stable, but not much improvement. I would frequently go shopping on my lunch hour, just to have some pleasant time to myself. I could escape all my problems, even if it was just one hour. When I had a few minutes, I would research SPS online. My curiosity would not let me rest, I needed to find some glimmer of hope in finding a cure for this. I thought about the possibility of being surveyed at work for surfing the web, but I didn't care. My mom's welfare was important to me. My boss was very busy at work and I hardly had time to talk to her. One day she came out of her office and said to me, "Did I ever tell you my husband got Lyme disease?" I said "No." I asked her how he got it. She said, he got sick after they came back from vacation in Wisconsin. He had a tick bite and said he was always fatigued. I asked her if he was ok now. She said "yes, he's much better now. He is fine."

Then she said, "You might want to check if your mom has Lyme disease." I said "No I don't think so, she's been verified by Mayo clinic and her own neurologist confirmed she has an autoimmune condition." My boss said, "well, it's an idea, maybe she has it?" "Think about getting her checked." In my mind, I didn't think she had Lyme disease. When I looked up the symptoms of Lyme Disease on the internet, none of the symptoms matched my mom's. She had ridged muscles, was very stiff and could barely move. She was also continuing to fall frequently. Her GAD antibodies on her blood test were high, her symptoms matched SPS and I had accepted that as her diagnosis. I printed some material about Lyme disease and brought it home. My mom tried to read it with a magnifying glass but she was losing her vision and that was the concern at the moment. I just hoped the surgery would go well.

I sat in the waiting room with my uncle Paul. My uncle brought a crossword puzzle to work on and I watched TV, but the whole time I was praying that my mom would be alright. Dr. Kay finally came out of the operating room and said her surgery was successful. We left the hospital and while she was in the backseat of the car, she kept saying she could not see right and started to panic. I said, "Mom, it will be okay, your eye is still adjusting." I took care of my mom for a few days at home and then asked an old friend of hers if she could help out until she was better.

A few months after the surgery my mom fell again. I was really concerned, not only that she would injure herself, but also disrupt her eye surgery. I hired another caregiver to help her at home.

At work, things were changing fast. A new healthcare law was passed in congress and I wasn't sure how that would affect us. In my department, leadership was changing and I felt more stress than ever. My boss was under pressure and my diabetes was out of whack. I wasn't paying much attention to my diet and I constantly needed a sweet reward. I was keeping candy and potato chips in my desk drawer. My weight started to go up, as well as my blood pressure which required medication. I had many sleepless nights and still tried to function like nothing was happening. I started to adjust to the new team at work, but they weren't the easiest to deal with. I was constantly bombarded with instant messenger on my computer and I had to leave my desk several times a day just to clear my head. I had to accept life for what it was – this was my new normal. There were a lot of meetings going on with my boss and all the senior executives. I began to get suspicious and my boss was blocking a lot of meetings as private on her calendar - something was up. I continued to call my mom at home several times a day to make sure everything was alright.

At this point I knew there would be a major reorganization going on and I kept thinking about headcount. There were several meetings scheduled on my bosses' calendar, one after another in her name. I realized they were calls about lay-offs. I didn't think too much about them, except this time, one of the calls was meant for me. I went to lunch that day, and then my boss came to me and asked me if I was on the call. I said I went to lunch. She said, "You were supposed to be on the call." I looked at her in bewilderment and said, "I was?" I realized I was one of the employees that was being laid off. I felt my heart drop into my stomach and my hands turned cold. Anxiety quickly turned to anger. My boss knew I was going to get laid off. After 13 loyal years working for her, she couldn't have told me herself? I was really angry. My mom was not well and now I was losing my job.

The next day, Human Resources had emailed me some documents to look over. Eight hundred employees were being laid off just in my department alone. I received a list of employee titles and ages of those being laid off. All types of roles were being eliminated with employees ranging in age from mostly their 40's to 60's. Some employees were lucky to be able to retire with the company package. I was not one of them. I had just turned 52 years old. The company offered the affected employees one month to look for another job internally, however if we could not find a position, we would not get an exit package. I decided to take the package. I knew it was a sure thing and I would get six-months salary and six-months COBRA to cover my insurance. September, 2013 was my last month with the company. I had so hoped to retire there, but that was never going to happen now. At least I had the exit package, which would last a little while.

My mom was distraught and she told me to take a break and look for a job in a few months. I agreed because I knew I could stay home and take care of her. Maybe this was a blessing in disguise. That same week I was invited to a get together with some of my old high school friends. We started talking and I told them I had been laid off from my job. One of the girls asked me if the lay-off was due to the new health care law. I told her I thought so. It was the older employees, who were more vulnerable to health problems, that were laid off. The company probably wanted to save the money they were paying out for health insurance, and I certainly fit into that category.

It was around 11:00 p.m. and everyone started to leave. I got in my car and turned on the radio where they were discussing a conference coming up at the local college about autoimmune disorders. The announcement kept repeating over and over, almost as if it was telling me to write down the website. I frantically looked for a pen and a piece of paper in my purse. There would be doctors from all over the world attending this conference and I wrote down the information. I went home and excitedly told my mom about what I heard and I asked her if she would like to go. At first, she said it would be too hard for her to function with the walker and sitting all day. I tried to convince her that we would be able to find something out about autoimmune diseases like SPS and a possible cure. She knew she would struggle, but she decided to go.

When it was time to go to the conference, my mom struggled to walk to the building with her walker. It was difficult for her, but she was a trooper and made it through the day. During the conference there was a doctor that spoke who told her story about how sick she had been due to several illnesses throughout her life. At one point she almost died, but then she started on the new treatment and returned to wellness. She mentioned she had lupus. My mom was also diagnosed with that. During the break, we waited in line to speak with her. My mom asked her if she would be able to treat SPS. She said "As a matter of fact, I just started treating a patient with SPS at my clinic and he is doing very well." We asked for her business card and her clinic was in California. She said "Come and see me, I think I can help you." My mom had a smile on her face because she was happy at the thought. She shook her caring hand. Could this doctor help her get rid of her autoimmune disease? We went back to listening to the conference, and they mentioned help for pain relief, autoimmune diseases, including diabetes, vitiligo, and multiple sclerosis. As I sat next to my mom, I said "we need to see this doctor in California." When the conference was over, I spoke to some of the other doctors, including one from England who said he had a patient with good results after treating his vitiligo. I wondered if this could help me. I then spoke to another doctor from Pennsylvania. He asked me how I heard about the conference. "Well", I said, "I heard you advertise on the radio of course." He said, "we never advertised this on the radio." I said, "are you sure, because I heard it advertised on there?" He said, "Positive. This conference was not advertised on the radio." My mouth dropped open. How in the world did I hear it so clearly and insistently advertised on the radio? I could only attribute it to divine intervention. I kept thinking about this conversation months after this conference.

After the conference ended, my mom and I were excited that there might be someone who could possibly get rid of her autoimmune condition. We had several conversations about going to see the doctor in California. Money was going to be tight, but I had to find out if my mom and I could get help. My mom agreed and I made arrangements for the flight. I ordered a wheelchair for transport to and from the airplane. It was going to be a challenge since she could not move without a walker and her fear was still there. I prayed to God to help me with this endeavor. When we traveled in the past, she could walk and carry her own suitcase, but now it was all on me.

In November, my uncle drove us to the airport. The airport was bustling and I asked an attendant to help with the wheelchair. I had to keep an eye on the suitcases and my mom. Finally, the attendant arrived with the wheelchair. She helped with putting some of the baggage under the wheelchair and my mom tried to help by holding some things on her lap. The attendant started to walk very fast and I had to pull my suitcase as well as walk briskly, almost running. I was exhausted just getting to the gate. The flight went smoothly and we arrived in California. The doctor's clinic was one half mile from the airport.

The following day, we had orientation with the staff at the clinic. We were going to stay three weeks for the wellness program. The first visit was routine testing, then doctor Dee, the one who we'd met at the conference, did an evaluation of all my mom's symptoms. When she first looked at the top of her head and saw her sores, she immediately said, "You are very toxic." My mom had red patches on her scalp which had been present for over a year. She also observed her skin was grey and she was very thin, along with the rigidity in walking and the obsessive fear. She had lost a lot of hair. Dr. Dee immediately ordered a comprehensive blood panel, urinalysis, heavy metals panel, allergy test, and a test to check for Lyme disease. I said, "Dr. Dee, my mom did have a tick bite in 2009." She asked where we lived, "Do you live up north?" "Yes", I said, "Near Wisconsin. We are actually not too far from the border." Dr. Dee said "We are going to see what the results tell us, but I don't suspect you have Stiff-Man Syndrome. I want you to start on the treatment for the auto-immune in the meantime. The medication works on the cytokines in the system. The test for Lyme disease takes about three weeks to process." Dr. Dee then asked me why I enrolled in the program. I told her I was having a lot of intestinal issues, infections, vaginal yeast infections, and thyroid issues as well as vitiligo, a skin condition and recently had cataract surgery. She told me right off the bat my problem was yeast, it was fungal. She prescribed an antifungal for me to start and then to review the test results with her when they came back in a few days.

Dr. Dee put both of us on a strict diet while we were at the clinic. No sweets or starch, mostly greens, specific fruits, and a lot of alkaline water. We were both prescribed; IV vitamin C drips, glutathione drips and hyperbaric oxygen treatments. We had shared meals everyday with other patients and talked about how we were feeling. I noticed how my mom's face was getting color back after four years following the oxygen therapy. I knew something was working.

During our stay, almost every meal triggered diarrhea for my mom. She had to go to the hotel room and rest frequently between treatments. I felt this might have been making her feel worse and not better.

The test results came back the following week and Dr. Dee reviewed them with my mom. She said my mom had extremely low levels of white blood cells, red blood cells and platelets. She also had a very high response to antibodies for Lupus. After hearing her report, it seemed like my mom was dying. How could this happen? How could her blood counts go so low like that? No wonder she felt like she did. Dr. Dee said the toxicology report for heavy metals indicated she had high levels in her body that included, mercury, cadmium and arsenic to name a few. Her allergy test came back with dozens of indications for allergies to all kinds of food with red meat listed as most severe. Her body was a real mess.

Dr. Dee recommended several supplements as well as a green powder drink for detoxification and another powder to heal her intestinal lining. She had leaky gut. She also recommended a sleep apnea test be done while she was at the clinic. When the test results came back, the apnea was very severe. She stopped breathing for 20 seconds between breaths. It did not surprise me at this point. Let's add another item to the list.

The doctor also reviewed my lab results. My thyroid levels were low and she advised me to increase my dosage and switch to a non-synthetic medication. I started on that right away. My hormones were also low so I started on natural forms of Estradiol and Progesterone. My allergy test came back with 15 mild food allergies. Dr. Dee also recommended a test that measures the health of the cells. I was told that my cell age was that of a 70-year-old, despite my being 52. It didn't surprise me as I always felt like I had low energy. After the evaluation, I started taking the specific supplements and natural medications my body was asking for. I started to feel a little better while I was at the clinic. The third week at the clinic was coming up fast. It was the week of Thanksgiving and they were serving us a real Thanksgiving dinner with turkey, mashed potatoes, salad and of course, apple pie! It was a welcome treat after being on such a strict diet. All the patients spent the afternoon with the doctor who owned the clinic, and discussed what we were all thankful for. I shared I was thankful to be alive after almost 50 years of diabetes and being able to help my mom recover from her illness. It was the best moment of our trip.

It was time to go home. We would have access to Dr. Dee for a year via phone as needed. We still didn't have the results back from the Lyme disease test for my mom, but I didn't think my mom would be positive for it. We had gained important knowledge at the clinic of what to do for better health. My mom started back on the IVIG treatment along with the additional supplements Dr. Dee prescribed. I started on the new thyroid medication as well as the others and supplements. My intestines were still not in the best shape, but I figured I needed time to see a difference.

About two weeks after we arrived home, I was aware that we had never received a call from the clinic about my mom's Lyme disease test. I called and they said they didn't receive the results. I said "Are you sure it's not there? It's been about five weeks." They searched and couldn't find it. I had a copy of the order that I brought home with me.

I called the laboratory myself and they told me the Lyme test results were sent to the clinic several weeks ago and they would fax it again. That same day Dr. Dee phoned my mom about the results. I looked at my mom's face as she was talking to the her. She had a wide-eyed confused look in her face. I asked "What is she saying?" She told my mom she didn't have SPS. The results came back positive for Lyme disease. My mom's expression was one of relief. Maybe now she would be able to get treated and cured. I was so angry about the doctor that failed to give my mom antibiotics for her bug bite back in 2009. Now everything came together – all the symptoms, the bite, the misdiagnosis. I was beside myself and didn't know what to do. I wanted revenge. All the experiences made sense now. She had pathogens in her body that were causing all these horrible symptoms which had affected me and my health very negatively as well.

Dr. Dee said mom would need to start on some oral antibiotics which she prescribed along with detoxification. We would need to locate a local Lyme literate doctor in the area. My new quest was to get my mom the help she truly needed.

2014 was a brutal winter. I got on the internet to search for physicians that treated Lyme disease. This was going to be a challenge combined with managing her diabetes. As I started to search for doctors, a local choice seemed impossible. However, I felt a 40-mile trip one-way in the relentless winter was too dangerous. She stayed on oral antibiotics until we could see a Lyme doctor in person. Little did I know that this disease would nearly wipe us out emotionally and financially.

As the winter passed, my mom had taken several rounds of antibiotics that upset her stomach and intestines terribly. She did not notice much relief from her symptoms or feel any better, and it was imperative to get the treatment she desperately needed.

May came and I was very anxious to get her to this Lyme doctor. I didn't want to see her in misery anymore and hoped this suffering could come to an end. The Lyme disease specialist was an older physician. He used to deliver babies, but after his wife and daughter came down with Lyme disease, he opened up a holistic center to treat it. He ran several tests on my mom to confirm Lyme disease and it was positive. First, he started her on IV antibiotics and a very strict diet void of sugar. The stress of the IV therapy and diet made her lose even more weight. Her diabetes was not controlled well. Along with the antibiotics, she also received vitamin C drips. The veins in her arms were mostly collapsed from the unnecessary IVIG treatment so it was quite a challenge to find a good vein on her arms. I drove my mom 80 miles round trip every other day for nearly three months to get treatment which was costing almost $3,000.00 per week. Insurance did not cover it because there was no such diagnosis as chronic Lyme disease according to the Center for Disease Control. By the time the summer was over, she spent over $30,000 and had to access important savings. It was ruining us financially. I could not hire anyone to take care of her since I had no income coming in myself. All I wanted was for her to recover. She was feeling a little better from the treatments, but she still could not walk without assistance or a walker. She still had high anxiety and unsteadiness. The cost for the infusions became impossible.

That fall I began to look for some options and a caregiver support group on the internet. Caring for my mom was a full-time job. I had no time to focus on my own health, no outlet for joy and everything was a crisis or a problem. I felt like the walls were caving in on me.

One evening as I searched for caregiver support groups, I discovered a new protocol for the treatment of Lyme disease. I clicked on the link and a doctor posted a video, including some testimonials from people who had recovered almost 100%. This protocol also treated autoimmune Type 2 diabetes, and even COPD. The doctor who invented this was also a scientist. He knew his stuff.

The next day, I told my mom about the website with new excitement. She said if I thought it would work, she was willing to try it. The testimonials of people that suffered with Lyme disease symptoms matched my mom's. Some of them had been completely debilitated and couldn't walk at all. Their before and after videos were remarkable. I also saw a few people that recovered from Type 2 diabetes. I contacted their office to find out more about the treatment and learned that it would cost close to $20,000. They would send a special formula and would tailor the treatment to specific symptoms. My mom said "Well there is still a little money left, this would be my last shot at something. Let's go for it."

I believe that in my deepest hour of need, God had directed me to this website.

My mom started on the treatment which consisted of a specific alkaline diet and a proprietary solution spray delivered orally followed by an oxygen treatment. I had a new role as caregiver, keeping tabs on the notes, vital signs, progress, webcasts and various supplements. With my background, it fit me perfectly. After daily treatment for approximately one month, my mom started to feel 50% better. She even stopped using the walker in the house and was moving around independently. I gleefully told the doctor she was making a recovery after five years of suffering. It was incredible and we continued on for another two months.

I started to apply for jobs because we desperately needed the money and I had to pay for my own health insurance because my COBRA benefits had run out.

An employment agency contacted me for a one-month assignment. I jumped at the chance, even though the hourly rate was half of what I used to making at my previous corporate job. The job was 10 minutes away from home, so I would be close by if my mom needed help. I was very anxious and I was taking a chance leaving my mom at home by herself. I taught my mom how to turn off the oxygen machine which she used every morning after the oral administration of the solution spray.

The first week on the job was training and since I had been unemployed for so long, it took a while to learn all the specifics. It was a stressful first week. The second week, as I settled in, I started to have an intermittent stabbing pain in the right side of my upper back. I sat quietly and tried to figure out the symptoms, as I tried to be cool and not raise attention. I timed the pain and I knew that if it was a heart attack, it would come on rather quickly. I didn't want to bring attention to myself and I knew I really needed the job and the money. They would find a replacement for me right away if I left. A co-worker had asked me to take a break and walk around for about 5-10 minutes. I was still having the pain, but I tried not to show it on my face. I couldn't wait to go home. The pain subsided a little bit, but it was still there, and I didn't mention it to my mom.

The following day I went to work, still having the pain. I figured I just strained a muscle in my back. That evening I came home and took a shower and when I looked in the mirror, to my horror, I saw raised red bumps like blisters on my right breast. I thought about shingles. My grandmother had it and she was in agony for weeks.

I got on the internet right away to find out how to treat shingles. I typed in diabetes and shingles and they recommended going to the emergency room immediately. I hesitated for a moment, because I thought there were other options. This could cause serious damage, even making my diabetes worse. It was time for action. I checked into the emergency room and the nurse came in to look at the bumps. She looked at it and said, "looks like shingles, but the doctor will be right in to check it." He came in and confirmed shingles, wrote the prescriptions and said I would not be able to return to work for at least a week. Not good news. I just started this job after a year of unemployment. This is all I needed! I had to explain to my employer and they said I could return to work when I was better. They knew that shingles could be contagious. I was hoping I wouldn't be let go, but at the same time I couldn't work with this anyway. The stabbing pain in my back was getting worse and worse. I started the medication and went to bed. The pain medication kicked in and I was able to sleep. The next day, I took the medication again and the pain killer. About an hour after eating I became very dizzy and felt like I was going to pass out. I told my mom, but she had her own issues and I wasn't sure how she would react. She said "I'm calling the paramedics." I thought I would faint at any second. I sat on the couch until the paramedics arrived. I sat back and closed my eyes. In about a minute, the paramedics were at the door, all 5 or 6 of them. They came to me and started asking one question after another. "What meds are you on?" I pointed at the bottles on the table. "Lucy" they said, "Don't fall asleep, try to stay awake." They started tapping my face so I would stay awake. They said they were going to put me on a stretcher and take me to the emergency room. When I arrived, the same doctor saw me in the emergency room. I had experienced a reaction to the pain killer and I decided I was going to skip any pain medication and just take the anti-viral for the shingles. I laid in bed for a couple of days in terrible pain without pain meds.

Prior to getting shingles, I had met with a holistic digestive expert. I emailed her to tell her what happened. She explained that she was going to mix various strengths of alkaline water, and that I should soak the sores several times a day with a washcloth. Amazingly, the sores started to go away and healed without a trace of being there. After the pain started to subside, I contacted my employer to see if I could return. I saw my primary care doctor who wrote me a return to work note. When I came back to work, I still didn't feel 100%, but I didn't want to forgo this opportunity for income. I was able to catch up and ended up getting extended for another month on the job. Ultimately it took several months for me to recover from the shingles. I constantly needed to rest and felt residual pain. At the same time, my mom was experiencing ups and downs while continuing to treat the Lyme disease.

In June I got another temporary assignment for three months. I would be working for a healthcare company that provided vascular services. The RN manager took a liking to me right away and appreciated that I had a medical background. The pay was a little higher for this job, so I was glad that I could finally make some more money. I had to leave my mom at home alone. Since she was starting to feel better, I thought she could handle being by herself for at least eight hours. I had to teach my mom how to fill in her vital signs and symptoms daily online. She was catching on quick and even learned how to attend a webcast. I was so proud of her!

The job was going well, and I had to get used to being flexible wherever I went to work. The manager said she would like me to eventually join the company as a full-time employee. I would then be eligible for benefits, including health insurance. My mom was concerned that the job was farther than I used to drive and was worried how I would get to work during the wintertime.

As the months passed, one-third of my paycheck was going to pay for mandated health insurance. That did not include the deductible that I had to pay before anything was covered at 80%. It seemed like all my money was going to pay for gasoline, health insurance and my medical plan deductible with very little left over.

Upon the decision-makers return, I sent an email to inquire about a full-time position. They said they needed approval from the CEO and they would let me know. They finally got the approval, but then I saw the contract and it was a per-diem offer with no guarantee of benefits. They also lowered the salary and at that point I was more upset than happy. I took the offer and stayed for a few months and then resigned. The job didn't have a secure future for me.

My mom was happy to have me back at home. While I was working, she had fallen again several times. This really scared me to think something more serious could happen while I was gone so I stayed home with her through the winter. My mom was slowly improving, but she still had set backs. This was not an easy disease to heal and it would take some time since we were taking a holistic approach.

Since I didn't have a steady job at the time, I lived on my savings until another opportunity came up. The same temporary agency contacted me about a position at a technology company. They were looking to add a role which would go from temporary to permanent after three months. I jumped at the chance because I needed a steady job with health insurance. I told the recruiter I would be interested in the position. She set me up for the interview with the employer, I was hired, and would start in a week. The first few days of the job went well, but then I woke up needing to rush to the bathroom and I felt very sick. I couldn't miss work, so I ignored it and went back to work. They had a staff meeting that day and I just sat in the conference room in total agony. I tried to look attentive and interested in the conversation, but on the inside I felt like a vice was attacking my abdomen. I felt relief when the meeting was over. I ran to the ladies' room.

Even though I was not feeling well through the course of the training, I still managed to learn many new things and I started to get quicker and more productive. My intestines continued to bother me for several weeks. I decided to get some tests which came back positive with several organisms; pseudomonas aeruginosa, staphylococcus aureus, and E coli. The very "bugs" I used to study in my college days years back. All I could think of was that my immune system is weak and now everything is attaching itself to me. Maybe a healthy person could fight it off, but with diabetes it is a whole different ballgame. The holistic digestive specialist put me on a whole bunch of remedies I was to follow for several months. I started on the new protocol and continued to go to work trying to meet the three month goal. I started to feel better and could get through the day with only minor problems. I knew the pseudomonas infection was a nasty bug and it would probably take a while for it to completely go away.

My mom was doing better at home, and there were no major incidents while I was at work. She attended the online webcasts with her doctor and told me they were opening up a location in the Caribbean to see patients in person. She asked me if I could take her there to receive some specific treatments for Lyme disease. I told her I had to make this new job work and develop into full-time with benefits. She frowned and I felt guilty about it. I didn't want to use up any more of my savings to pay for health insurance and I rejected the thought of going on Medicaid.

The second month I was on the job, the recruiter came by to take my boss and I to lunch. The recruiter had told me that my boss was very happy with my job performance. I thanked them and said I looked forward to staying with the company. I gave a sigh of relief, something good was on the horizon.

I came home and told my mom that the lunch went very well, and I had one more month of work to qualify for the permanent position.

The very next day, there was a big management meeting at work. Afterwards, I got a call from my recruiter. She said they were cutting temporary workers due to a budget crisis and I was affected. I was at loss of words at this point. This had happened over and over, and I began to wonder if I would ever have a job again. I was asked to pack my things and leave within the hour. Out like a piece of trash, a day after I was told my job performance was great. I wanted to cry, but that would only get me upset. They walked me to the door and I gave them my entrance ID tag and went home.

Once again, I had to tell my mom I had some bad news. She couldn't believe I was out of a job again and I immediately told her we would be able to travel to meet her Lyme doctor in person. Maybe he could also help me with my intestinal issues while I was there. My mom and I talked over the trip. It would be incredibly expensive and yet I knew it was worth it if her recovery process could be improved. We would stay for a month, and my mom would get all the treatments she needed.

The following week we went to a travel agency and made arrangements. The day of travel arrived and I was as anxious as could be. This would be an international flight, with one stop in Miami before we arrived at our destination. My mom was a trooper. She got through the aisle helping to carry some small bags, although I kept looking behind me to see if she was okay. She still had a huge problem with anxiety from the Lyme disease. The doctor planned to meet us at the airport and we would drive to the clinic together. We got buckled in our seats and then we waited on the tarmac for an extra hour, which was unexpected. I kept hoping we would not miss our connecting flight. When we arrived in Miami, we only had 10 minutes to get to the gate. My mom got on the airport vehicle and I ran to the gate to tell the flight attendant we were there to board. I had three bags with me and the gate attendant told me they only allowed two. One bag had all my insulin pump supplies and I was told I needed to check it. I said, my medications were in there and I could not afford to lose that bag. She argued with me and said I needed to give up one bag, and I had no choice. Mom and I boarded the plane. We had the last two seats left!

We arrived safely and my suitcase with the insulin pump supplies arrived as well. We had help with the bags, and my mom was given a wheelchair. The doctor was waiting outside and he yelled out my mom's name. He recognized her and gave us both a hug and a kiss. It was a very warm greeting from a doctor I knew was genuine and special. He cared about his patients healing. The ride to the clinic was long and bumpy but scenic. We saw some very beautiful scenery and stopped for some barbecued chicken along the way. We were both very hungry from the flight. We arrived at the hotel and settled in. We stayed right on the shore and it was a nice get away from our stressful lives back home. The next day would be the start of my mom's treatments and she couldn't wait.

The staff prepared three meals for us every day. They kept our diets alkaline based because this supports faster healing, especially with the Lyme disease. Bacteria thrive in an acidic environment. The first week my mom started to learn to walk in the pool. Her doctor who also had a background as a physical therapist, helped her in the water to get her to balance and eventually she learned how to float and then swim a bit. It was incredible. I didn't think she could do it, but I was very impressed. She also received light therapy on a weekly basis and ultrasound along with other modalities. The area had some steps along the mountains near a waterfall. Mom started to climb stairs by holding on to the rails. The atmosphere was helping her tremendously. Eventually, the doctor took her for a walk on the beach without her walker for about an hour.

The staff at the clinic were all very friendly and extremely helpful. One of the staff members carved a cane out of walnut for my mom, to graduate her from the walker. They also let me use one of the treatments to get rid of my intestinal infection. He had mentioned I could also probably get rid of diabetes, but I couldn't afford to continue after the trip. Our trip was coming to an end and my mom said she felt about 80% better. I was getting excited and I felt better too.

We arrived at the airport to go home and had to go through customs again. The attendant scanned my suitcase and then brought me through the electronic scanner. My insulin pump triggered the scanner. The attendant approached me and said "What are you wearing?" "I wear an insulin pump for diabetes," I said. "Ohhh", she said with a long sigh. "Oh my dear girl", she said. She had such compassion on her face and I figured she must have had some sort of experience with diabetes. I told her a bit about my experience. "Oh, I'm so sorry," she said. She told me many people on the island also suffer with diabetes and that people die from it without much knowledge or proper care. I felt more compassion from that one woman, then from almost anyone I knew. It was a heartfelt moment.

We arrived in Miami and had to wait for an escort to get us to our gate. A very nice and good-looking man came with a wheel cart to take us. We had tried to tell him where we needed to go, but he had a hard time understanding. He spoke little English, but fluent Spanish. He and my mom spoke in Spanish to get clearer directions on our flight time and gate. Everyone from our flight, plus other arrivals were waiting in front of us. At this point, I was getting nervous. We had to get something to eat. The diabetic woman that was escorting us, said "Don't worry, they owe me a favor," and she was able to get us closer to the front by cutting in line. My mom started to have a low blood sugar episode while waiting in the line. She had nothing in her purse except some pretzels.

The TSA agent said she couldn't put anything in her mouth. The diabetic woman escorting us said, "she needs to have something or she will faint, she is a diabetic." The pretzels helped her to get through the line. I was paranoid the whole time thinking she could faint. The woman escorting my mom hurried to get us through to the touchscreen to enter our information. Millions of people must have touched this with their hands every day. We were in such a hurry, that I had to get through all the screens fast before it was accepted. We got the printouts to take to another station. They checked our photos with our passports. After that, the woman took off with my mom in the wheelchair, and I ran struggling behind, pulling my purse and two suitcases. My mom asked where I was, and the woman said I was right behind them, but in reality, I was about a block further behind.

When we arrived at the gate, I thanked the woman and told her to take care of her diabetes. She was so wonderful for getting us to our gate on time. They were already boarding our flight and fortunately there was a food vendor next to the gate. I bought two bread rolls and a couple of turkey sandwiches and carried the bag of food along with the suitcases. I was so overloaded. My mom tried helping by pulling her suitcases through the aisle. I was exhausted by the time I got to my seat.

I got settled, took out my glucose monitor and started testing my blood sugar. It wasn't too bad, about 130 mg/dl. I was very happy I didn't have a low blood sugar during that whole ordeal. The woman sitting next to me asked me what I was doing. I said "I'm checking my blood sugar, I have diabetes." "Oh," she said, "Yes I know what diabetes is, my husband is a chiropractor." I then took out my insulin pump and my sandwich and started eating. I didn't even get a chance to wash my hands before getting on the flight. I ate the sandwich and then felt like it just wasn't moving down my intestines, just sitting in my stomach. The woman next to me kept talking and joking around, but I was just too exhausted to care. I was just hoping I didn't need to use the restroom mid-flight. Both passengers next to me watched me eat. I settled into the seat and then just kept watching how much longer the flight would be. We arrived and I couldn't wait to get home to rest.

My uncle Paul was waiting for us to bring us home. When I got home, I unpacked a few things and ate some leftover meatballs from the freezer and a can of peaches. Shortly thereafter I went to bed. Around 1:00 a.m., I needed to rush to the bathroom, I got up and fainted. I don't know how long I was passed out. When I regained consciousness, I realized I was on the floor with my knees buckled and my head in the corner next to the toilet. I felt awful and couldn't stand up. I crawled into the hallway with my arms and yelled "Help Mom!", "Help", but she was asleep. I crawled through the rest of the hallway and with much agony got up on my bed. I used the cell phone to call my mom on the land-line phone to get her to wake up. I told her I had fainted and I was all sweaty. She called the paramedics and they arrived in less than five minutes. When I was in the ER, they checked my vitals and my temperature was 101 degrees, but I was not dehydrated. They said my urine PH was alkaline and the nurse told me I took good care of myself. They did a urine culture and would have the result right away. I tested positive for an E. coli infection. The ER doctor put me on antibiotics and anti-parasitic drugs, and I was to take them both for one month. The month following, I was in complete agony in my lower intestines. I felt very tired and could barely do anything. I definitely had something "bad", I just didn't know what it was. I just prayed day to day that each day would be better than the previous and I could recover. My mom was doing much better after the treatment in the Caribbean. She went to her primary doctor and told him, "I feel like something was lifted from me." I felt great for my mom, but now I was in tough shape. My mom had a bit more energy and was walking without a walker in the house. I was so happy that after six years, she was beginning to return to normal.

About a month later, my mom was in the kitchen cleaning up after lunch. She started to tie up the garbage bag, bent over and took a slight turn in her step. In a flash, she started falling forward, fell on her left wrist and hit her head on the kitchen counter. I started screaming, "Mom, are you alright?" She was dazed and shaken from the fall. She said "I twisted my wrist." It looked swollen and I said "I'm going to call the paramedics." She said "No, I don't want to go to the hospital." "Okay", I said, "The wrist feels hot, I can't determine if it is a sprain or a break. I'll wrap it in an ace bandage." I looked at her head and there was a scrape and a bruise. I cleaned it with hydrogen peroxide and put an antibacterial cream on it. She was doing so well. Now that she'd fallen again, I was so worried I didn't know what to think. My own health was compromised again and I had this new set of concerns. I begged her to let me take her to the orthopedic doctor, but she refused. Now she returned to using the walker.

My health continued to worsen. I couldn't handle more of my own problems, as well as my mom's. It was just too much for me. I spent several months in agony with my intestines. I couldn't even bother to look for a job and bills started piling up. My mom's treatments were costing a lot of money and I couldn't get well enough to do anything about it. I had no choice but to apply for Medicaid, something I absolutely hated the thought of. I never in my life wanted to be on public aid and be a burden.

The presidential election was coming up and I decided to write a letter to the new candidate. I wrote some action items for him to consider and the importance of encouraging the medical profession and scientists to seek cures for chronic conditions, such as diabetes and Lyme disease.

In the beginning of 2017, Mary Tyler Moore had passed away. My diabetic idol was gone. I felt like I lost a soul sister. I always imagined that maybe someday I would get to meet her, but that day will never happen. I can only imagine how she suffered as well.

I continued to struggle with my intestinal issues. With alternative treatments, I was starting to feel a little bit better. My mom was still not feeling as well. I found out she did indeed break her wrist and she continued to have anxiety and pressure headaches. The winter months went by and I continually looked for doctors in the local area that could treat my mom.

When spring arrived, I began taking her to new doctors, but then experienced another attack with my intestines and got very sick again. I was afraid to get dehydrated and end up in the hospital. The diabetes control was up and down, and my blood sugars were out of whack. I was still in no shape to look for a job.

My mom spent time on the phone with her friends and was told by a friend of hers from church that there was an alternative practitioner that would be able to find out what my issue really was and help my mom with her Lyme disease. We made an appointment. The new doctor had technology that could evaluate what was happening in my body by placing my hands on a metal plate hooked up to the computer. It would read what was going on internally. When she started to go through my intestinal system, there was evidence of several amoeba's, parasites and flukes. I also tested positive for H. pylori, Giardia lamblia, E. coli and several other waterborne parasites. I had never determined how I got sick after coming back from the Caribbean, but now it was confirmed. I also was quite surprised that on the computer scan it also showed that I had insulin independent diabetes – Type 2. I said "I have Type 2 diabetes?" with surprise. My thoughts were on a spark collision. Wow. Could this be true? The doctor said, "Yes, you have Type 2. This could be corrected with some gluco-balance tablets." I didn't believe it. I already had experienced 53 years of diabetes, how could I possibly reverse it? I started thinking back, and for many years I was only on one injection per day. Most Type 1 diabetics need more than one injection per day to survive. Could I have been misdiagnosed with Type 1 diabetes to begin with? I put the thought out of my head and said "Okay, let's treat my infections first." The doctor had me do some treatments on the computer to do a detox and then kill the infections with light therapy. It took several months of this treatment before I started to feel a little better, but I was improving. My mom was also checked with their technology and it was confirmed that the Lyme disease was in her brain. She started treatments as well.

I found myself wondering about the type of diabetes I actually had. Could my diabetes have been caused by some sort of virus or pathogen that destroyed some pancreas cells when I was a small child? Could that virus or pathogen still be encased in my pancreas and living there? I thought about the virus that causes chicken pox and how it can hide many years in the nerves of the body and then be triggered once again many years later to come out as shingles in an older person. Is there something holding my pancreas back from its full function? After over 50 years of living with this condition, will there ever be a cure in sight, or even a cause established?

With diabetes every day it takes focus and willpower to be a "good diabetic." Like most diabetics who take their condition seriously, I try to follow the diabetic diet guidelines and yet, my blood sugar can still escalate. It's a daily commitment to accept the relentless requirements of managing diabetes and hoping to outlive any serious complications.

There is still an uncertain future with diabetes. How much longer is the wait for a cure? There are diabetics from all walks of life that share in my silent solidarity. Together we are as one battling on for survival and hope that one day, we will all have a chance to be finally free from diabetes.

In the interim, self-care and vigilant management of our diet and overall wellness is the absolute best thing we can do for ourselves. Learning the art of acceptance is essential and making ourselves available as support to each other enables making the best of each day.